DISCOVER
ESSENTIAL OILS
FOR OPTIMUM
HEALTH

Other Books Published by HieroGraphics Books LLC

"12 Week Dream Journal"
Julia L Wright, editor

"Monthly Dream Journal"
Julia L Wright, editor

"Gratitude Journal"
Julia L Wright, editor

Handbook To Health
Vivian Rice and Edie Wogaman
Revised and edited by Julia L Wright

Where Do I Belong?
Susan Grace

Galloping Wind: The Legend of Wild Shadow, The Wind-That-Gallops
Zoltan Malocsay

Sinister Frog
Bob Kelsey

**Natural Health Book Series Based on
Orison Swett Marden's *"Cheerfulness As A Life Power"***
Available on Kindle, Revised and enhanced by Julia L Wright

Book 1: Laughter and Essential Oils:
Natural Cures for Dis-Ease

Book 2: Optimism and Essential Oils:
Natural Cures for Depression

Book 3: Positive Attitude and Essential Oils:
Natural Ways to Alleviate Stress

Book 4: Cheerfulness and Essential Oils:
Natural Ways to Create a Joyful Life

Book 5: Giving and Essential Oils:
Naturally Create the Life You Desire

Book 6: A Sunny Nature and Essential Oils:
Naturally Create Optimum Health

As A Man Thinketh
by James Allen
Revised and enhanced by Julia L Wright

**For more insights on ways to fall asleep naturally,
live a holistic life or create abundance in your life visit:
www.HolisticSteps.com.**

DISCOVER ESSENTIAL OILS FOR OPTIMUM HEALTH

An Essential Guide for
Using Essential Oils
to Naturally Achieve
Your Optimum Health

****

Holistic Steps

****

Julia L. Wright

Published by HieroGraphics Books, LLC
First Printing, February 2012
Second Printing, February 2016

Printed in the United States of America

HieroGraphics Books, LLC
106 Ruxton Ave
Manitou Springs, CO 80829

www.HieroGraphicsBooksLLC.com

Many thanks for the loving knowledge imparted
by my teachers, healers and friends
who helped create and edit this book

Judie Gephart
Kathleen Morrow
Despina S. Struck
Roger Tolzman
Vivian Rice

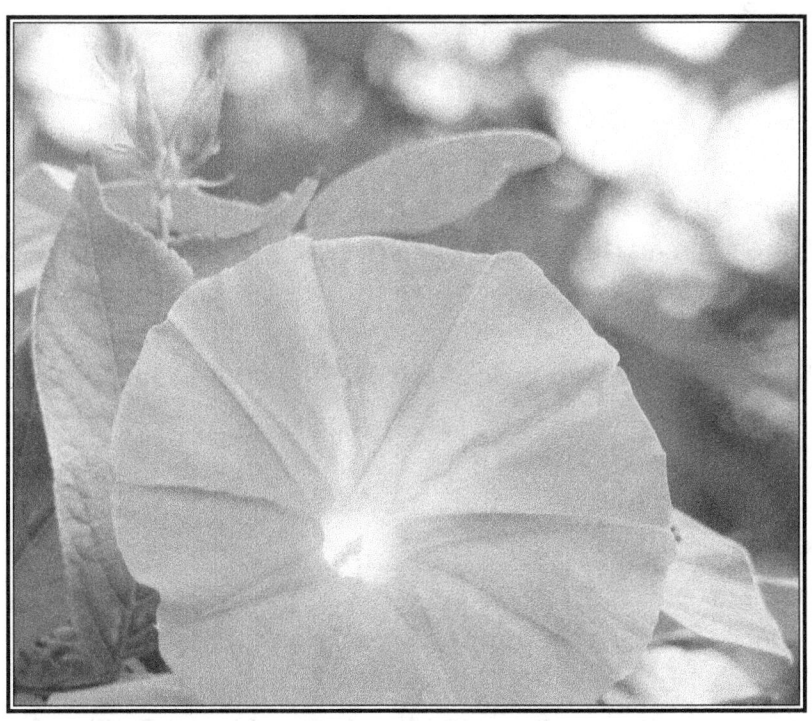

"Healing is embracing what is most feared;
healing is opening what has been closed;
softening what has hardened into obstruction;
healing is learning to trust life." *Jeanne Achterberg*

INTRODUCTION

Dear Reader,

For over 19 years, I have used essential oils for a wide variety of purposes aiming at bringing optimum health and abundance into my life while protecting the environment.

I have used essential oils for healing my body and mind; cleaning my home; relieving pain and emotional stress; for spiritual support; and preventative health care. You can cook some essential oils to add zest to favorite recipes. Others you may add to hot or cold water to create healthy, refreshing cold drinks and soothing warm teas.

Over the years, I have shared many of these tips and bottles of essential oils with friends and family members to help them through times of emotional challenges or a physical health crisis. I have encouraged them to enjoy the pleasant aromas or tastes to help cheer their day and heal their bodies.

Here you can discover the unique qualities of over 50 essential oils and how to use them for specific purposes.

I have found that using therapeutic-grade essential oils makes all the difference when looking for specific results regarding health issues.

Be sure to always use 100% pure therapeutic-grade essential oils for healing or massaging into your body and when ingesting or cooking with essential oils.

Immediate Benefits

Often, when you begin to use essential oils, you will begin to see and feel the benefits immediately. Sometimes it takes a bit more time. Usually when using them for aromatherapy to change a mood, the results happen within moments after taking in your first deep breath.

I know you will enjoy these ideas and find this book an interesting read. Visit my blog at www.HolisticSteps.com to maintain your optimum health using essential oils and other steps.

I would like to encourage you to try any essential oils that interest you to discover your optimum health.

NOW! is the time to take your first step towards improving your physical health and / or mental attitude with a safe, natural method that has been used all over the world for many centuries.

Important Information Below
About This Book - Please Read.

The information found here is for educational purposes only. This book is not intended to diagnose, treat, cure, or prevent any disease. It is not meant to be a substitute for medical care or to prescribe treatment for any health conditions.

This book was written for people who are seeking natural, non-toxic, non-addictive, chemical-free wellness ideas and are willing to actively participate in gaining optimum health for themselves and their families.

Not all of these Tips will work for everyone, but all have worked either for myself or a friend or ten, who have written or told me about their positive results they have experienced from using essential oils.

May your Life Always Be Filled with
Peace, Joy, and Optimum Health.
Julia L. Wright

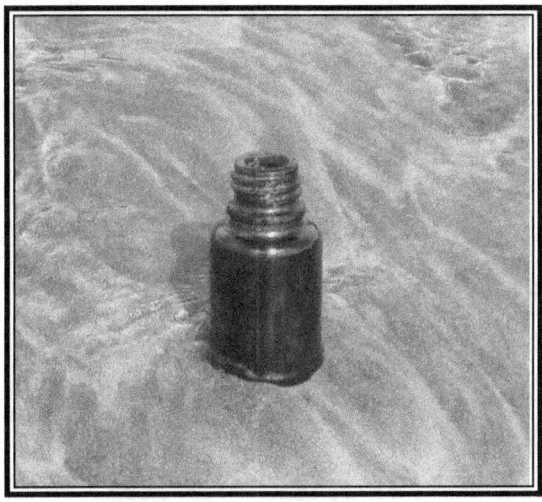

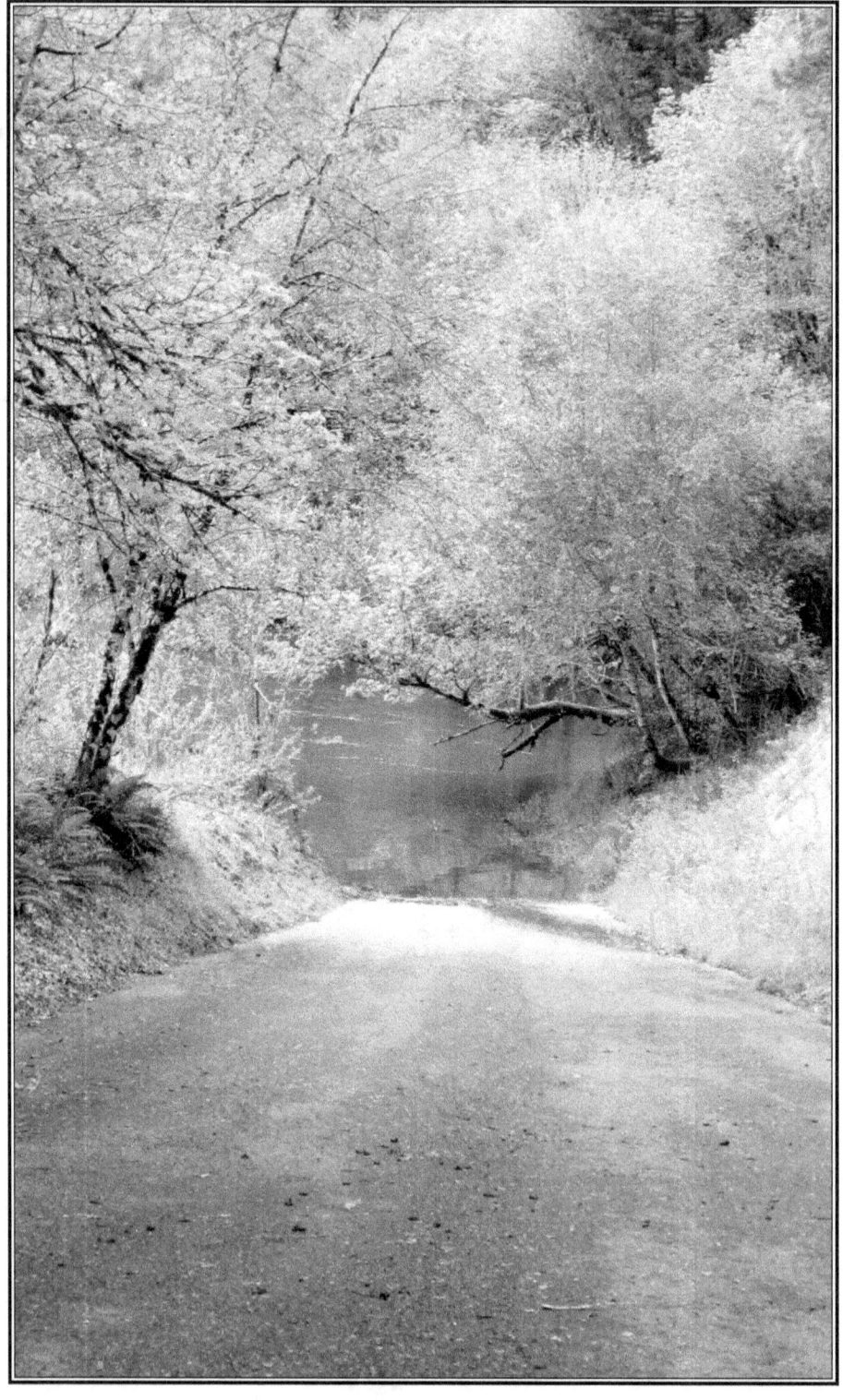

CONTENTS

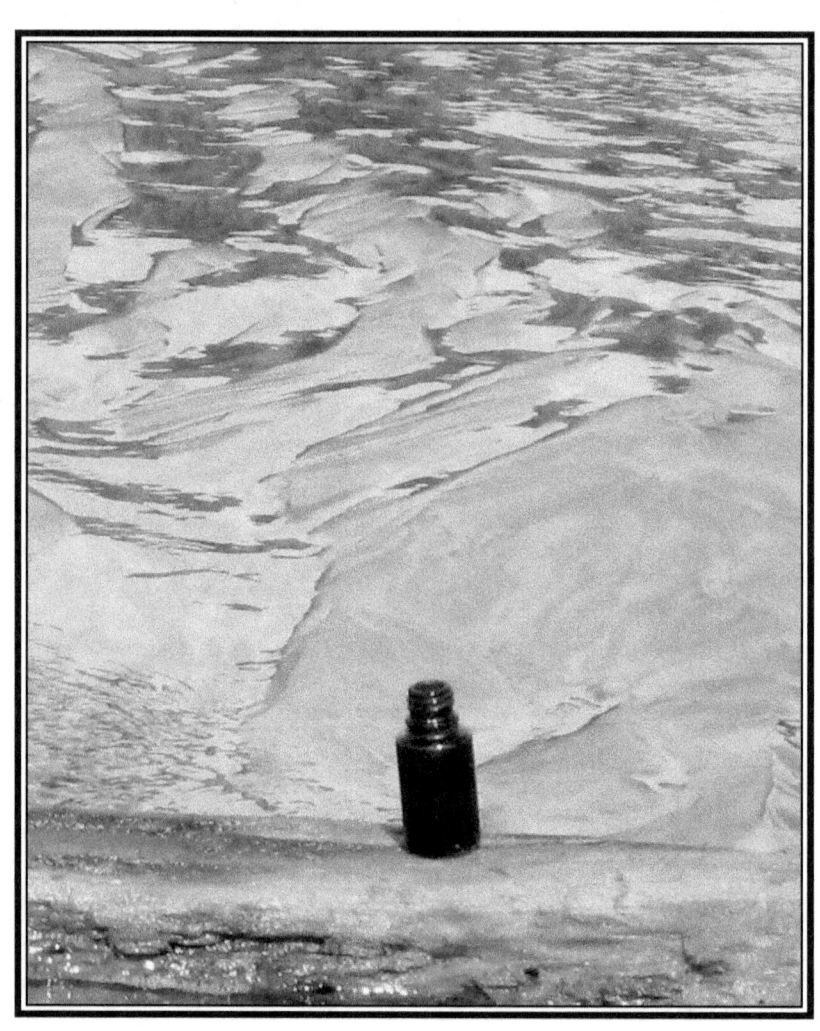

Chapter 1

WHAT ARE ESSENTIAL OILS?

Perhaps you have been intrigued when you have heard some friend talking about "essential oils", but don't understand what they actually are, where they come from or how to use them safely.

Throughout history and in every civilization around the World, essential oils have been used for cooking, perfume, beauty aids, massage, aromatherapy and medicinal purposes.

Nature offers these amazing healing gifts found inside all plants that can be used to help heal the body, clean homes, uplift a spirit and enhance the flavor of any food.

Essential oils are more potent than dried herbs. When you use essential oils, they often yield faster, longer lasting results when used as natural remedies for health challenges than if you used dried herbs. A single drop contains a very potent distillation of each plant's healing energies.

All plants contain complex and powerful substances that we have defined as "essential oils".

Each has one, or more, specific properties that can be used for various purposes to live a more naturally healthy life.

These distinctive components are referred to as the "essence" of the plant and they determine its aroma.

Some of these essential oils are easier to distill and access than others. Aromatic liquids can be derived from different parts of a variety of types of plants.

A distillation process is used to distill essential oils using flowers, trees bark or resin, roots, bushes or shrubs and seeds. Different companies use numerous methods of the distillation process. Different methods will create much more pure oils than others.

Modern research shows that 100% pure essential oils can provide many natural health benefits for humans and animals experiencing health challenges or just want to enjoy a more natural way of living.

Essential Oils vs Imposters

There is a huge difference between therapeutic-grade 100% pure essential oils and less expensive copies that may have been produced in a lab using chemicals or have been diluted with alcohol.

It is imperative to chose high-quality essential oils to gain positive healthy results and not chance creating a new health challenge.

Essential oils differ in chemical composition from other herbal products because the distillation process recovers only the lighter phytomolecules. This is the reason essential oils are rich in monoterpenes and sesquiterpenes, as well as other VOC substances (esters, aromatic compounds, non-terpene hydrocarbons, some organic sulfides, etc.)

There are many products on the market that claim to be *"essential oils"*, but when you read the labels you will notice they may contain an essential oil, but they are often diluted with alcohol or other products.

Any fragrance product other than therapeutic-grade 100% pure essential oils are not recommended to be used in any healing process to avoid creating new health challenges.

Some of the added ingredients in other products can actually irritate a person's skin when massaged on the body.

These adulterated *"essential oil"* products most certainly should never be ingested or used when cooking.

Essential Oils Popularity

Essential oils have recently experienced a huge revival as natural, safe and effective products to help resolve many types of health challenges, clean homes and aid minds to be more relaxed and happy. Essential oils can be used as one step to create a more holistic approach to your life.

Essential oils can now be found in massaging products and topical pain relief and medicinal compounds. Always read the ingredients used in these products!

Make doubly sure they are using only truly natural, 100% pure essential oils and don't contain any other ingredients you can not easily pronounce to avoid irritating your skin or causing other health challenges.

It is preferable to purchase the essential oils or oil blends that have properties that you require relating to any health challenge you wish to address.

You can then add a few drops to a pure carrier oil, such as olive oil, when applying them topically. Or put a few drops into rice milk or olive oil when ingesting essential oils. This way you know exactly what you are putting in your body and don't have to worry about ingredients that may take away from the healing properties of the essential oils, or even cause an unwanted side-effect.

Essential Oils Around the World

In many countries outside the United States, essential oils are included in the national pharmacopoeia.

On the European continent the use of essential oils is often incorporated into mainstream medicine. It is not unusual for a doctor in a European or other countries around the world to "prescribe" an essential oil to resolve a person's health challenge.

In many countries, the use of the antiseptic, antiviral, antifungal, and antibacterial properties of oils are used as a way to control infections. Their use is often emphasized over the approaches familiar to North Americans.

In France some essential oils are regulated as prescription drugs, and administered by a physician. French doctors use a technique called the aromatogram* to guide their decision on which essential oil to use.

Many commercially available pain relief ointments include various essential oils in their ingredients giving validation to the healing properties of these elements.

People around the world have repeatedly bought millions of dollars of these essential oils, so it must be assumed they have helped them to feel better naturally in many ways.

Properties of Essential Oils

Each essential oil can be used for one or more health challenge and in one or more ways to create health for you and your family.

Different essential oils are recognized as valuable for having properties that can be used as natural approaches to common health challenges.

Below are listed some of the most common properties that essential oils have:
- Calming
- Uplifting
- Energizing
- Focusing
- Relaxing
- Digestive Aid
- Decongesting
- Cleansing
- Hormonal Aid
- Antiviral
- Antibacterial
- Anticarcinogenic
- Antifungal

* aromatogram (er·o·mat o·gram), *n.* a test used to determine the antibacterial activity of essential oils in which the oil is introduced into the center of a bacteria-laden petri dish. A clear zone indicates the bactericidal activity of the oil.
The greater the diameter of the zone, the higher the efficacy of the oil.
Definition provided by: http://medical-dictionary.thefreedictionary.com/aromatogram

Essential oils work in three different ways to achieve these effects and help a person gain optimum health:

1. At the scent level they activate the limbic system and emotional centers of the brain.

2. When added to massage oils and applied to the skin, they activate thermal receptors and may kill microbes and fungi.

3. When small doses are orally ingested, they may stimulate the immune system.

How Essential Oils Work

Through the use of essential oils, it is possible to gain access to wonderful therapeutic results.

Two basic mechanisms are offered to explain the purported effects when using essential oil aromatherapy for the treatment or prevention of disease. One is the influence of aroma on the brain, especially the limbic system through the olfactory system. The other is the direct pharmacological effects of the essential oils.

Although the benefits of alternative therapies like aromatherapy are not easy to prove or disprove, there are numerous encouraging results from scientific studies for a number of health issues. Scientific evidence for the healthy effects gained from using essential oils is both growing and still in the preliminary testing stage.

Even though aromatherapy as a science has never been recognized as a valid branch of medicine in the United States, Russia, Germany, or Japan, many preliminary clinical studies concluded in Europe and around the world have shown many positive effects when used to treat numerous types of mental, emotional and physical health challenges people experience in all walks of life.

Why Use Essential Oils?

When using essential oils you will experience no side effects, just pure beautiful natural energy released to change your life in many positive ways.

Maybe you have wondered how essential oils can be used to increase health naturally.

Or you may be wondering what is the best way to use specific essential oils to create the maximum healing benefits from each oil?

When traveling, would you like to have a safe and effective natural hand sanitizer?

Ever wished for a more environmentally friendly way to clean and sanitize your home?

Would you like an air and carpet freshener that doesn't contain harmful chemicals?

Have you searched for a natural way to gain energy?

Or fall asleep more easily at night?

Would you like a natural way to relive inflammation?

Ever wondered if there was a natural way to calm your nerves and find peace in a stressful situation?

Essential oils have many natural healing properties and may be the perfect approach to resolving health challenges, both physical and emotional, that you, or someone in your family may be experiencing.

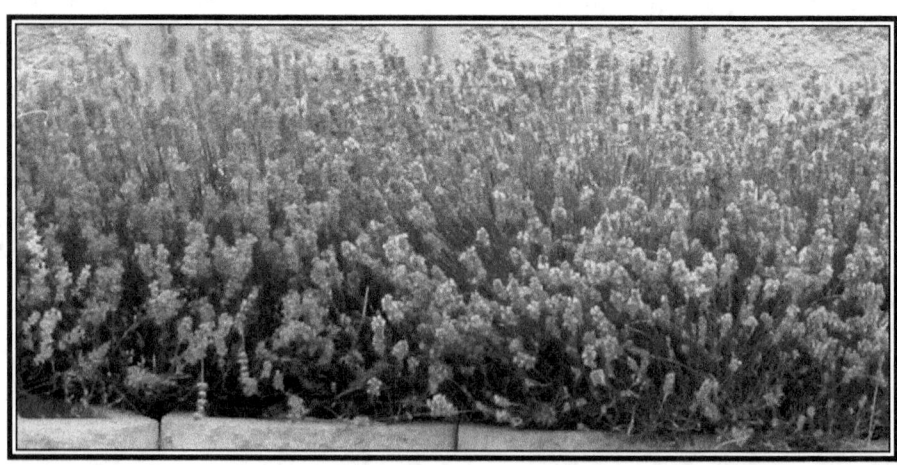

Popular Uses of Essential Oils

The two most popular and basic uses of essential oils include massaging them into the body or using aromatherapy and inhaling them.

Historically, medicinal and aromatic plants have been used to purify and scent places, scare away evil spirits, treat skin and other physical disorders.

Many cultures cook using essential oils rather than herbs for more powerful flavoring of foods.

Many Massage, Craniosacral, Reiki and Lymphatic Therapists use aromatherapy in their practices. The therapist may use a specific single oil or create a custom oil blend for individual client's specific needs during each visit.

A good therapist will ask questions about how you are feeling, any health specific concerns you may be experiencing and your emotional state at the time of the visit. Using this information, they will choose essential oils that can address your specific physical health challenges or emotional needs during your visit.

They often add the essential oils to a carrier oil, or they may place drops directly on your skin and softly massage the essential oils into your body.

While you are receiving a massage, you can deeply breathe in the aroma of the oils to help relax your mind and assist the oils to enter your system in two different ways: inhalation and topically.

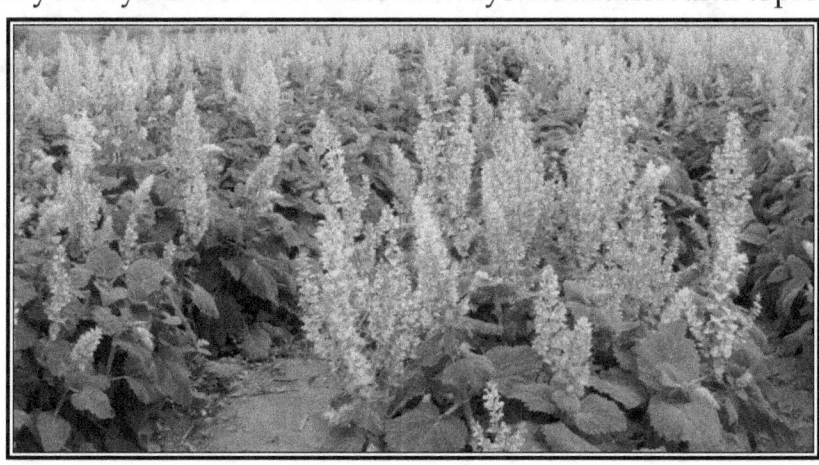

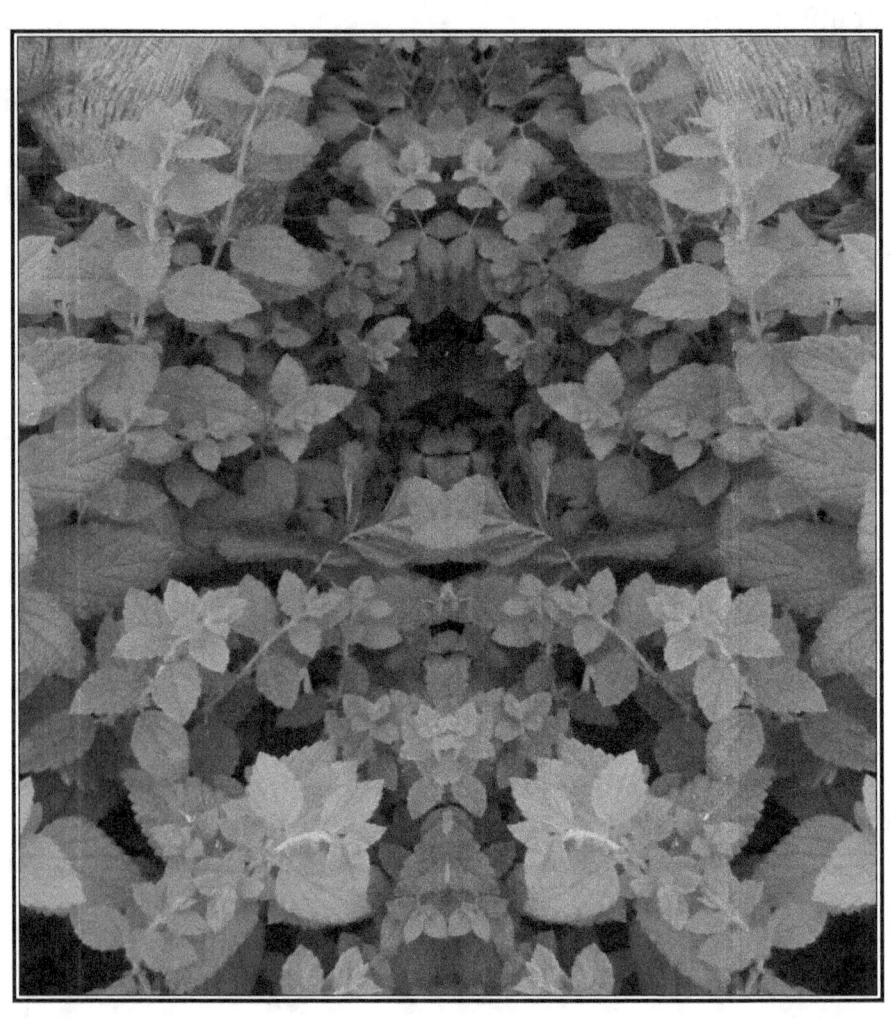

About Essential Oils Tips

On the following pages various essential oils are defined by their aroma followed by a description of some of the properties each essential oil is best known for in healing circles Worldwide.

After many of the essential oil definitions are *"Tips"* for ways to incorporate them into your daily life to help you regain or maintain your personal optimum health.

I invite you to take some time to read the following pages describing various essential oils to help you better understand how and why they should be used by you.

How to Share Your Essential Oils Tips

If you have some really good tips about how essential oils work for you and would like to share these with other people to help them on their path to optimum health, please email them, along with your name and city to:

info@usingessentialoilsforhealth.com.

Be aware that by sending us your tips and stories that you are granting us permission to publish them and post them on the internet in one of our blogs, as well as to edit them for length, mechanics and content.

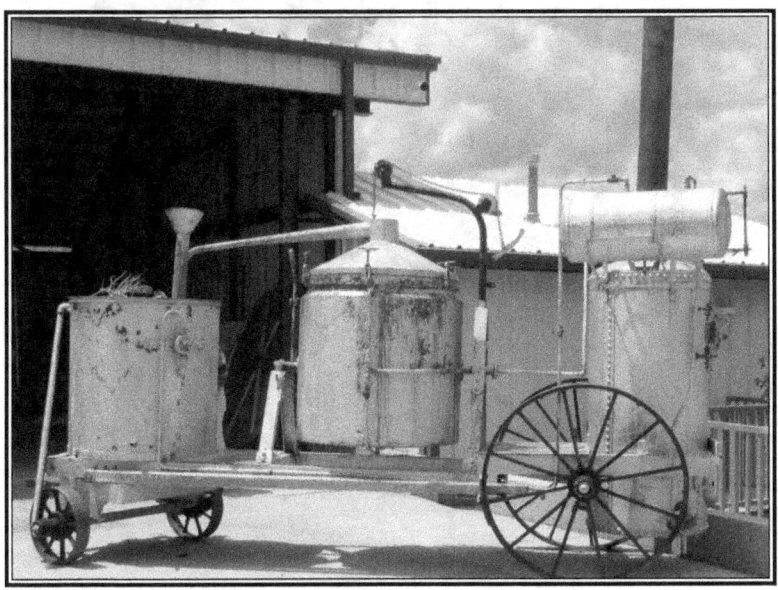

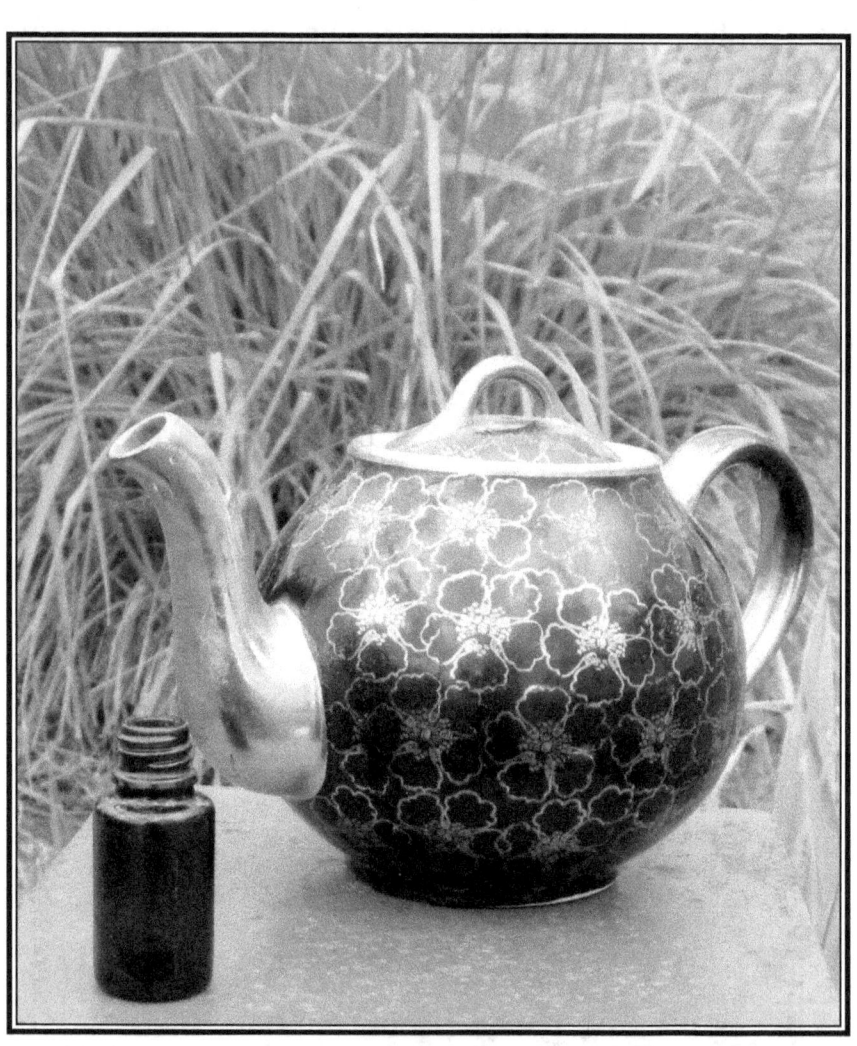

Chapter 2

THREE BASIC WAYS TO USE ESSENTIAL OILS

There are many ways of using essential oils as an important element to begin creating a healthier life for you and your family.

These are the three basic ways you can add essential oils into your life and journey to optimum health.

Each method works best for specific treatments to improve health or enhance your life.

Whichever way, or combination of ways you chose to use essential oils, be sure you are using 100% therapeutic-grade essential oils.

Lesser quality oils can actually create more health challenges than they would resolve.

Always test a small amount of a new essential oil before ingesting, inhaling or massaging a larger dose on or in your body.

It is important to keep in mind that everybody's (everybody's) tolerance is different.

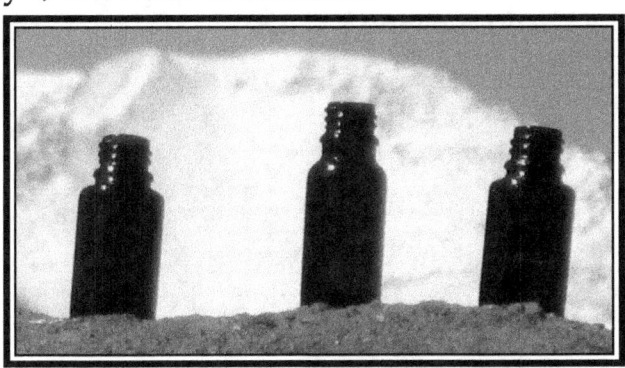

INHALATION
(OFTEN REFERED TO AS AROMATHERAPY)

Inhalation of essential oils heightens the senses and different scents can trigger many desired responses in the body, mind and emotions.

One of the most popular ways to use essential oils is by inhalation, also referred to as aromatherapy.

Here are just some of the many ways to get the benefits of using essential oils for aromatherapy:

1. Simply smell them from the bottle or cap. Move the bottle away while exhaling to keep the bottle as pure as possible. Or use alternate nostril breathing while inhaling from the bottle.

2. You can add essential oils to bath water. When adding an essential oil to your bath water, it is best to add the essential oil to a pure liquid soap or bath salts, then into the water–it disperses/emulsifies better than adding directly to water.

3. Use a special tea-light candle burner underneath a ceramic small bowl filled with pure water. Place a few drops of essential oil in the water. It will then vaporize into the room. Using a candle or heat to diffuse will provide aroma, but may alter or damage the healing properties of the essential oil.

4. Essential oils can be diffused using a variety of commercial cold-air diffusers. This is the best method for diffusing essential oils for healing purposes.

5. Fill a humidifier with water and place a small cloth that you have sprinkled a few drops of essential oil on in front of where the steam exits.

6. Carefully pour hot water into a small bowl. Add a few drops of essential oil. Cover your head with a towel. Lean over the bowl, breathing slowly and deeply.

7. Place a few drops of an essential oil on a cloth or cotton ball and carry in a pocket or purse or place it under a pillow at night.

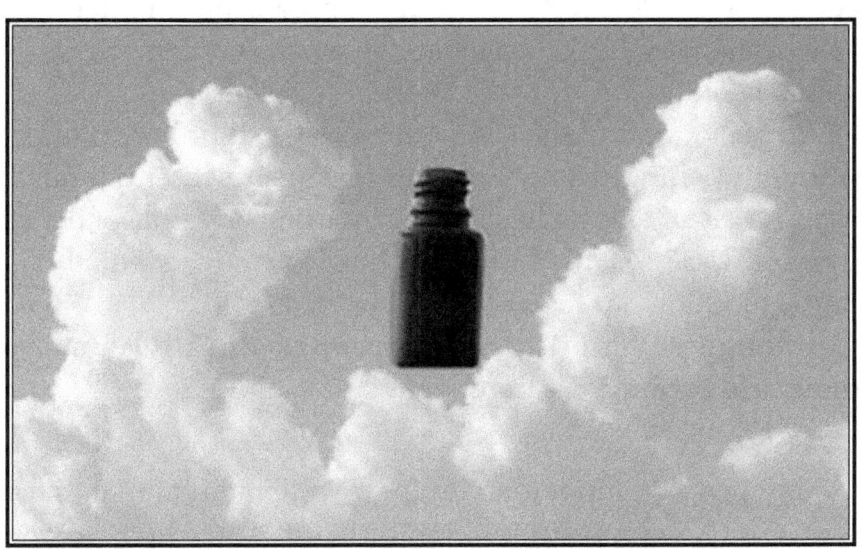

TOPICAL APPLICATION

Another popular way to use essential oils is to apply essential oils directly to your body and massage them directly into the skin.

Some essential oils are very potent and may cause irritation to the skin. With that in mind, it is suggested to test an area of skin with each new oil before applying more than a drop.

It is best to dilute essential oils for topical applications to avoid this problem. Diluting an essential oil with a carrier oil will allow a larger area of skin to be covered.

Dilute the essential oil using a pure vegetable oil or natural oil compound when massaging them into your skin. My favorite vegetable oil is a high quality, pure olive oil.

Be careful to avoid getting the essential oils or aromas to close to your eyes or in the inner ear.

ORALLY

Some essential oils are more effective when taken orally.

You should only use 100% pure therapeutic-grade or food-grade essential oils labeled as dietary supplements for internal use.

Rice milk, olive oil or water are the most common liquids used to dilute essential oils for safe internal consumption.

Add 100% food grade essential oils to cold or hot water for a healthy refreshing drink. Creating teas using essential oils is a delicious way to enjoy a healthy, warm drink any time of the year. See pages 32-33 for more ideas on how to enjoy essential oils to create a soothing hot tea or refreshing cold drink.

Although some oils can be dropped directly upon your tongue, use extreme caution here.

TEST!

Many people cannot tolerate spicy well and that makes using essential oils without dissolution difficult. Their lips, the tissue inside their cheeks and under the tongue are usually the most sensitive areas. When essential oils stay on the tongue and are swallowed without coming into contact with the other areas, many people experience minimal displeasure or discomfort from this method.

Dilution and dosage varies dependent upon the age, size, and health of each individual. **TEST!**

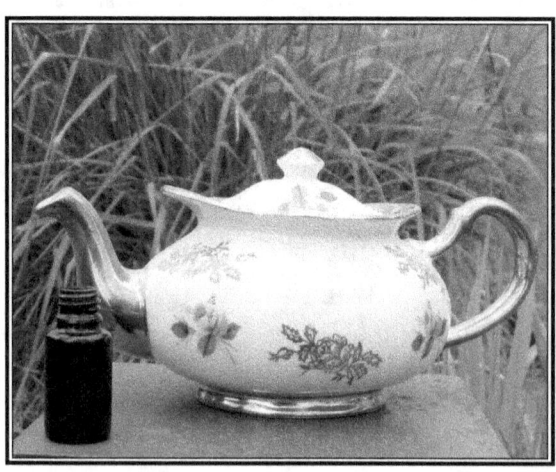

COOKING WITH ESSENTIAL OILS

Cooking with essential oils is another way to enjoy their healthy benefits. Using essential oils in place of dried herbs will add a stronger flavor to your recipes.

Adding oils while cooking can greatly enhance flavor. If you want to enjoy the healthy benefits of the oils, add after cooking when food is slightly cooler.

When using oils while cooking be aware that food-grade essential oils are very strong.

For instance: 1 drop of Young Living's peppermint essential oil has the same strength as 28 cups of peppermint tea! It is much stronger than in dried herb form.

When using food-grade essential oils for cooking sometimes even 1 drop of oil can create a stronger flavor than desired.

A good method of testing could be to put a drop of essential oil in the food–test the taste–then adjust flavor by adding more if you desire a stronger flavoring.

This is a good method to test the flavor, especially for stronger oils such as: oregano, thyme, basil, peppermint, etc.

"Once within your system, essential oils will work to re-establish harmony and revitalize those systems or organs where there is a malfunction or lack of balance. Their effects are many and varied, but they are noted in particular for their antiseptic properties and their ability to restore balance to both body and mind."

"A variety of factors help to determine the effectiveness of aromatherapy treatment: the quality of the essential oils, their appropriateness for a particular individual or a specific ailment, the methods by which they are applied and, in the case of a professional treatment, the extent and quality of interaction between the therapist and the patient."

from the book: Aromatherapy for Common Ailments by Shirley Price

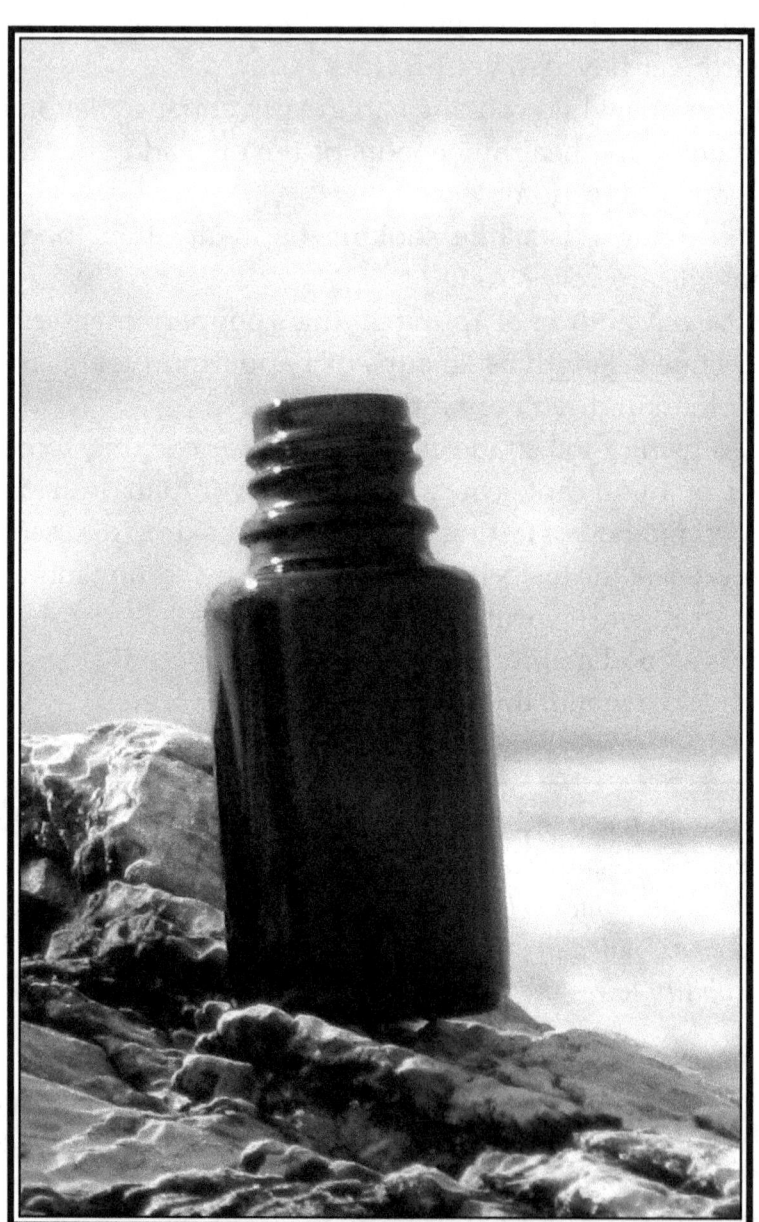

Chapter 3

WHERE TO BUY ESSENTIAL OILS

B e aware when buying any heath product, that some companies are more ethical than others. Be particularly cautious when purchasing essential oils to use for healing.

Not all distillation processes create therapeutic-grade essential oils. Not every company insists on using organic plants for the distillation process. There are even some companies that will add a only a couple of drops of 100% essential oil to claim their oil as pure.

Do Your Research Carefully!

There are many companies that can be found on the web or in health food stores that sell essential oils.

Some companies sell very high quality products, and some are more ethical than others.

There are some companies who will add chemicals or other oils to their product, so it is no longer a pure essential oil, more of a perfume quality product.

Some businesses are notorious for selling blends without identifying their ingredients.

Some of these companies give detailed information on how the essential oils are used, most don't. Be sure to ask questions to determine what all the ingredients are in these blends that they are selling. Are they really pure essential oils? Or are there other ingredients added? Where do they source the plants that are used to create the oils? Who does the distillation? These are other important questions to ask the seller of essential oils?

Ask Questions!

If you are looking on the internet, you might want to take some time to comparison shop. Notice the differences in the descriptions of the essential oils. Do they claim to be therapeutic-grade? How do they back up this claim? Where are they distilled? Where are the plants grown?

Prices can tell you a lot about the product. More exotic or rare essential oils, like frankincense or sandalwood, should have much higher prices. *If not, something is wrong.*

Check out seasonal sales. Some companies offer you free shipping when you order a certain amount of the essential oils or have annual sales during the year.

You can sometimes encounter individuals in your area who actually produce high-quality essential oils. There is a woman in my area that produces helichrysum and lavender essential oils from plants she sources from an organic grower creating an very pure quality product. My sister-in-law works for a company in Oregon that carries a few high quality essential oils. To find this type of quality in a small distillery is very rare.

Buying essential oils requires giving thought to what purpose you are using them for and taking some time to get the right quality for your needs.

Be aware that some essential oils may interfere with medications you are taking. ALWAYS consult with your primary care-giver before adding essential oils to your healing process.

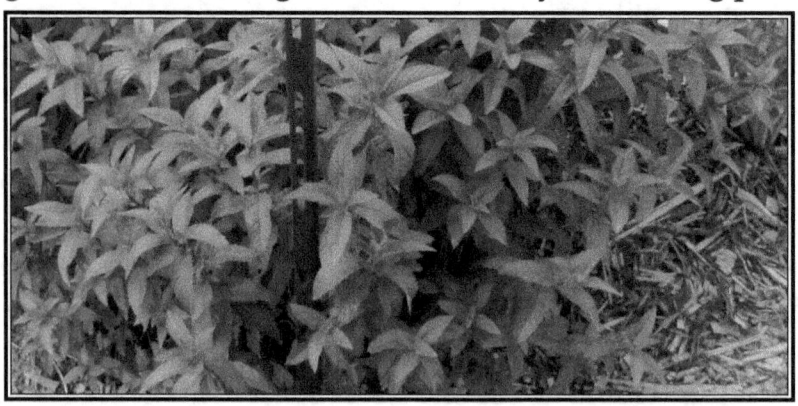

Julia's Favorite Essential Oils Resource

I have used Young Living products for over 19 years. The quality of the oils and the integrity of the company has convinced me that they offer the very best essential oils currently available.

Visit my web site: http://www.youngliving.com/juliaw

At this web site you can read more about essential oils, the company Young Living Essential Oils and their policies.

If you decide you would like to purchase some essential oils, you are invited to do so on my website.

Or perhaps you will decide you want to become a Young Living member/distributor so you can purchase your essential oils at wholesale prices and invite abundance into your life.

You may wish to help others by guiding them onto this healthy path with you and introduce them to Young Living Essential Oils.

If someone besides Julia shared this book with you, ask them how to work with them to learn more about essential oils and Young Living. If you have lost their contact information, check the first page on this web site to connect with them: www.usingessentialoilsforhealth.com.

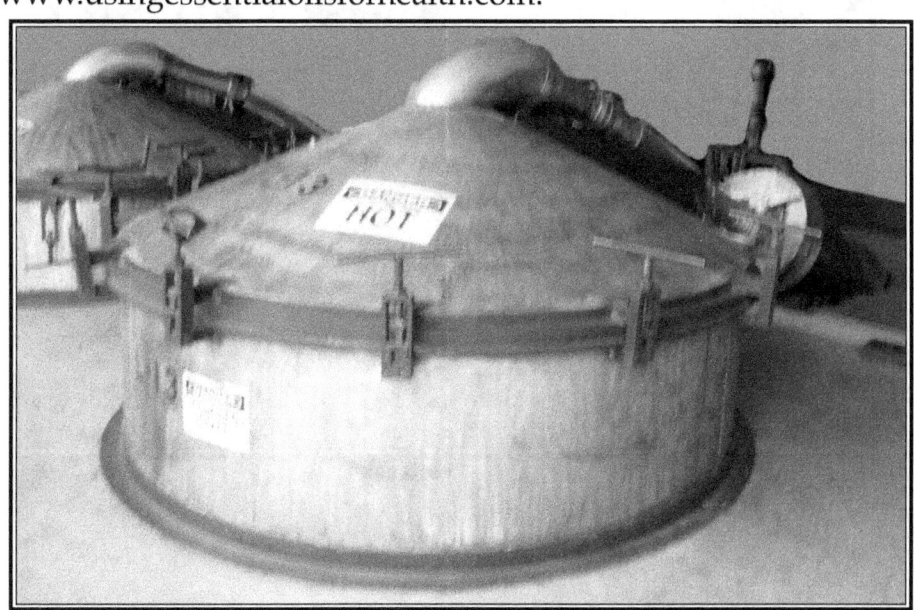

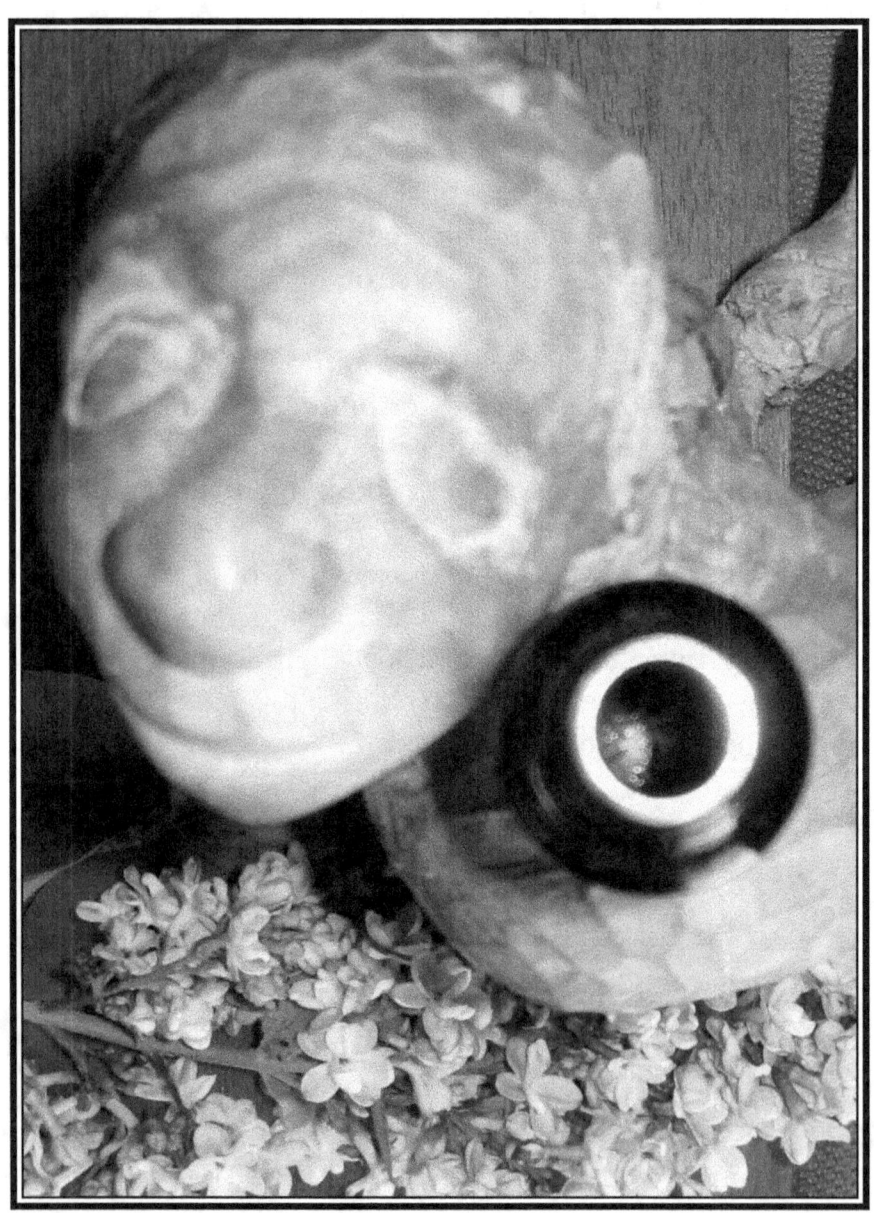

Chapter 4

WHERE TO START?

Three Versatile Essential Oils

If I had to chose only three essential oils to keep with me at all times, it would be these three extremely versatile essential oils: Lavender, Peppermint, and Lemon.

In this chapter, I share some of the easiest ways you can get started using the three most widely used and versatile essential oils to naturally enhance your life and health.

Each has a wide variety of helpful properties and can be used in all three methods that essential oils can be experienced: *Inhalation, Orally and Topically.*

Single essential oils and blends have a variety of uses to help promote a healthier life in many ways. The more you use essential oils, the more they will become a part of your home life.

I use a variety of essential oils EVERY DAY to keep me alert, brighten my mood, relieve stress, clean my home, ward off germs, help promote good circulation in my leg, relieve muscle aches and add pleasant, healthy scents to the air in my home and office.

It is highly unlikely for anyone to experience uncomfortable or unnatural side-effects when using plant-based pure essential oils to handle a health challenge. Many traditional solutions for health challenges can have unnatural side-effects. Often people may even find they are feeling worse when they use pharmaceutical solutions for even simple health challenges. Many just treat the symptoms, not the source, so they often don't solve the core health challenge.

Lavender Essential Oil

Lavender essential oil is often referred to as the Universal Oil. It is probably the most versatile essential oil and works in many ways to help a person experience mental, emotional and physical health.

There are many natural health benefits to be gained when you inhale, ingest, diffuse or massage areas of your body with lavender essential oil.

You can create a chemical-free air freshener by putting a few drops of lavender essential oil in distilled water in a spray bottle to spray around your home or office space. *(Inhale)*

Rub lavender essential oil on cuts or bug bites to reduce swelling and help them heal quickly to ward off infections. *(Topical)*

You can create a soothing tea by adding a few drops of food grade lavender essential oil in hot water. *(Ingest)*

Pure, therapeutic grade lavender essential oil can help to balance your energy in many ways. Although it may seem counter-intuitive that it can both relax and energize, it does.

Lavender essential oil has properties that will calm your mind, uplift the spirit, rejuvenate, relieve stress, energize, relax, comfort and revive both the mind and body.

The most common use of lavender essential oil is to help a person relax at night to help get a deep and sound sleep. Inhaling it as you prepare for bed helps to relax both your mind and body and soothes stressful emotions..

There are many essential oils used to uplift spirits, but lavender is the one aroma used by more people in various cultures around the World for this purpose. Lavender essential oil is used in many ways to balance moods. It is an adaptogen and can assist the body when adapting to stress or mental and hormonal imbalances.

Many people use lavender essential oil to relieve stress and anxiety. It is one of the best oils to use for relief of these problems when life seems exceedingly challenging.

If you experience stress without substantial relief for a long period of time, please consult with your primary health care giver.

However, you may want to try diffusing and massaging with lavender essential oil first.

Lavender essential oil has balancing properties, when inhaled and massaged on the body, can help relieve extreme stress. The calming aroma of this essence helps a person stay relaxed during stressful times and situations. Putting a drop on your heart area or under your nose when you are feeling stressed will help you feel relaxed and centered.

Although lavender essential oil is best known for its relaxing and calming properties, it can also be used to energize your mind and to help lift your body out of the feeling of being fatigued. When you feel more relaxed and less stressed, you will find energy returning to your body.

Lavender essential oil is one of the best essential oils to use for relieving headaches. Massage lavender essential oil on your temples and the bridge of your nose for relief from headaches.

Be careful to avoid getting the oil or its aroma in your eyes.

Take a moment or two and close your eyes and visualize a pleasant place to rest. Meditate on a peaceful image for at least five minutes for the best and fastest results.

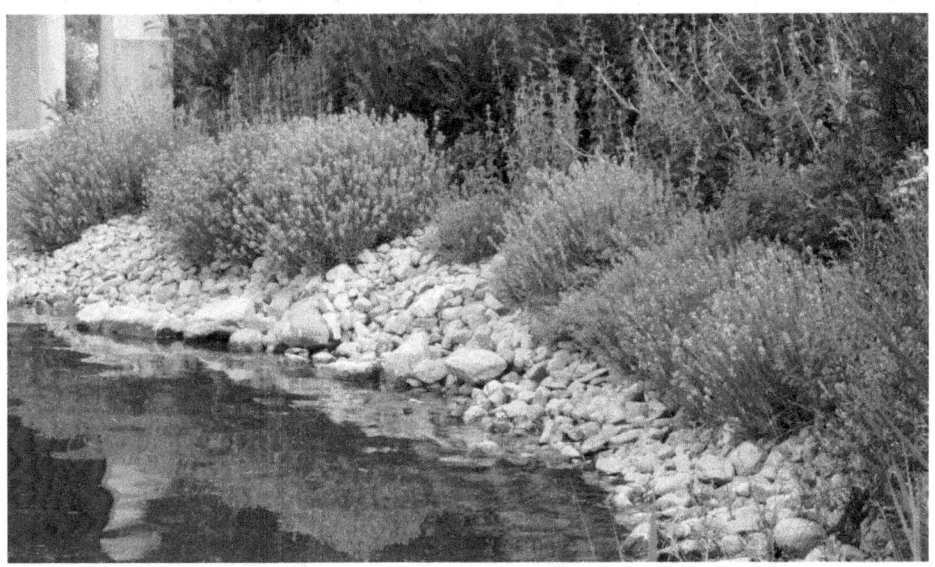

Lavender essential oil can be diffused to help reach a deeper, more focused meditation. Try rubbing a drop on your temples to deepen your experience when meditating. This helps to relieve tense muscles and let go of negative thoughts.

Women find its aroma particularly helpful to redirect negative emotions they experience PMS and during their menstrual cycles.

Keep a bottle in your purse. Open it and take in a few deep breaths of this soothing aroma when you find yourself feeling sad, angry, or stressed for no obvious reason. Its aroma helps bring you back to center and feel more like normal yourself again.

Lavender has antibacterial, antifungal, and antiviral properties, so it can be used to fights germs on skin and in the air.

Use it to help cleanse cuts, bruises, and skin irritations.

Its antibacterial and anti-inflammatory properties helps cuts and bites to heal quickly and avoid infection.

Use it to soothe minor burns by applying 2–3 drops of lavender essential oil to the affected area.

Lavender essential oil has antioxidant properties and supports the immune system. Spray or diffuse lavender essential oil in areas when you encounter other people who display signs of having a cold or the flu to help protect yourself from catching their germs. Inhaling its aroma directly, or using the diffusion method, may help your body defend itself against viruses and germs you come into contact with when around strangers during the day.

Do you realize that underarm body odor is most often created by accumulating bacteria? A natural way to stave off this problem is to use lavender essential oil. Place a drop on your underarms to keep odor down. If you are sensitive to essential oils, add a bit of lavender essential oil to a carrier oil before rubbing it under your arms.

A few drops of this highly effective antibacterial essential oil can be added to water to wipe or spray around bathrooms, kitchens, and sickrooms or any area you want to disinfect.

I like to carry it with me when I travel to breath while traveling on a plane or in crowded places. I put some on hankerchief and place it inside a plastic bag that I open often when traveling.

Lavender essential oil is used in massage therapy for relieving sore muscles and other body pain. Different kinds of pain can be soothed by using lavender essential oil. Massage it into sore, stressed or tired muscles to help relax these muscles and relieve the physical pain. When massaged into sprained, strained or pulled muscles, its anti-inflammatory properties help to keep swelling down associated with these types of physical injuries.

Lavender essential oil is highly regarded for creating healthy skin and radiant beauty. It can be found in many natural skin and hair care products. Throughout the centuries, lavender essential oil has been used in skin products for the entire body. It is especially favored for facial treatments to relieve dry and cracked skin; reduce wrinkles; and acne.

Although it may sound counterintuitive, essential oils can help to clear oily skin, people around the World have been getting good results using a rinse made from various essential oils, including lavender. Add a few drops to a small amount of water to use as a rinse for your face after you wash it. Put a few drops in a carrier oil to enjoy natural, gentle relief from dry and itchy skin.

Be aware that some pets dislike any aroma or have allergic reactions to them, just as humans do.

Yet, most pets are able to tolerate them, some are even drawn into the room when you are diffusing essential oils. And just as with humans, some essential oils can be a great help as natural healing solutions for a health challenge your pet is experiencing.

TEST! very cautiously when using essential oils with pets.

Always take extreme care when using essential oils on or around animals. Watch for any signs of distress in a pet when you first use essential oils around them. Take them outside or into another room if they seem uncomfortable around any oils you are diffusing or wearing.

Lavender essential oil is one of the few essential oils most pets can tolerate being used on their body and many actually enjoy this calming aroma.

Our grandmothers understood that lavender was a good way to repel insects. Try rubbing a few drops of lavender essential oil on your ankles, wrists and neck areas before going outside to discourage flying pests from landing on and biting you.

Placing some drops on a cloth or a few cotton balls in closets can help to keep moths from damaging fur, feathers and clothing. Lavender essential oil also helps to keep stored seasonal linens smelling fresh. Replace the cloth or cotton balls, or just add more drops, every month for the best results.

Besides being known for its medicinal qualities, food grade lavender essential oil has many culinary uses. Lavender imparts a delicate flavor when cooking with it. Lavender honey is a delightful addition to baking and teas.

Because it has so many health benefits, I truly believe that no home should be without lavender essential oil!

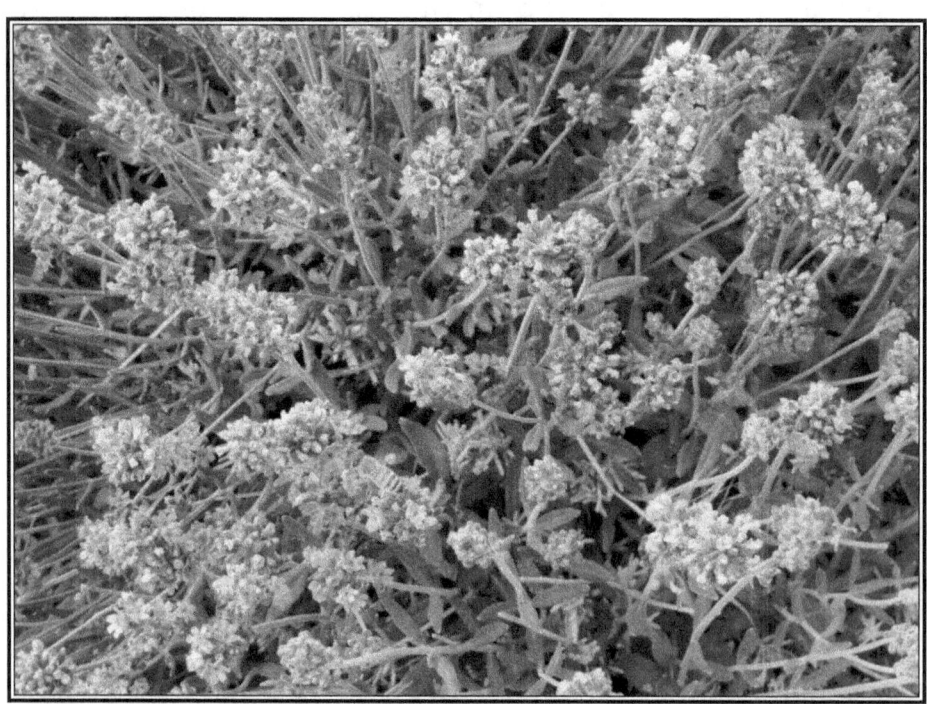

PEPPERMINT ESSENTIAL OIL

There are many ways that diffusing and inhaling or massaging the body with peppermint essential oil can create natural health benefits for everyone.

Take a deep breath of peppermint essential oil when feeling tired for a quick energy boost. *(Inhalation)*

Massage peppermint essential oil onto your temples, or on the back of your neck for relief from a headache. *(Topical)*

A drop of food grade peppermint essential oil a glass of water will create a drink that actually cools the body and is very refreshing, especially during the warm months. *(Ingest)*

Do you ever find it difficult to wake up in the morning? I know it can be a struggle to embrace wakefulness some mornings.

Caffeine doesn't agree with my nerves, so every morning when I want to feel more awake, I use peppermint essential oil.

Try this when you awake feeling groggy in the morning. Open a bottle of peppermint essential oil and rub a bit on the nape of your neck and below your nose. Next, take a couple of deep breaths in. Allow the scent to resonate in your brain for a few moments before you start your day. When you do this, you will find yourself feeling alert, wide awake and ready for whatever the day may bring. Use peppermint essential oil when you awake each morning to feel perky and excited to start your day and feel naturally energized all day.

One of the most important reasons I use peppermint essential oil is it helps keep me alert.

When inhaled, the stimulating aroma of peppermint essential oil helps improve concentration and increase mental sharpness.

If you are in a work situation and feeling tired or distracted, take a moment to inhale a bit of peppermint essential oil or put a drop or two in your water glass to give you an energy boost and bring your mind back into focus.

Keep a bottle of peppermint essential oil in your car. When you get in your car, put a drop or two under your nose. Breathe in its rejuvenating scent before you leave your driveway or drive home at night. This will help you stay centered and feel more focused on your own driving. Plus, you will feel more alert and that can help you to avoid problem drivers.

Do you ever experience bodily pain? Or, have times when you forgot to stretch your muscles before exercising, and then find yourself in pain? Are your muscles stiff and sore when you try to relax into sleep at night or when you awake in the morning?

Have you ever experienced a leg cramp? STOP! Don't reach for a bottle of pills, there's a better, more natural way to relieve aching muscles from the outside.

Peppermint essential oil is used by many people around the World to relieve aching muscles.

When you use peppermint essential oil you may find you won't need to see a professional massage therapist or use pharmaceuticals to find relief.

Place a few drops of peppermint essential oil in a carrier oil, such as olive oil. Slowly and deeply massage any areas on your body that feel stiff or sore. Most often, you can work out the stiffness of your muscles by yourself with a little help from peppermint essential oil. Soon you'll be feeling your spry self again; ready to hit the trail or courts; or run another mile.

Peppermint essential oil acts as a general stimulant when massaged or ingested to help bring your body back to its natural warmth when you are feeling cold.

Externally applied, can also give relief from the stiffness associated with rheumatism.

Do you experience headaches? Rub a bit of peppermint essential oil on your temples and the nape of your neck, being careful to not get it in your eyes. Take a moment and close your eyes and relax your whole body. Deeply breathe in its minty scent, soon your muscles will relax and the headache will disappear.

Taken internally, it may help restore digestive efficiency or help curb appetites. It directly affects the brain's satiety center, which triggers a sensation of fullness after meals.

To freshen your breath, put a drop in water instead of using a sugary after dinner mint.

If you have an upset tummy; or have eaten a new food causing your stomach to feel queasy afterwards; or have eaten too much heavy foods at a party and came home feeling bloated, you need natural relief for these stomach ills.

Nature has many herbs that can help relieve an upset tummy without creating another unnatural side effect, that can be sometimes caused by using pharmaceutical products.

Pure, food grade peppermint essential oil is one of Nature's best solutions to help sooth minor digestive discomforts. To relieve an unsettled stomach and aid with digestion after any meal, put a drop in some water and sip it to calm your stomach. Or you can apply it topically to ease a queasy stomach. Add a few drops of peppermint essential oil to a natural carrier oil, like olive oil, and rub it onto your stomach area to get quick relief.

**I would suggest every home should have
a bottle of this wonderful essential oil on hand
to naturally help relieve a variety of health challenges.**

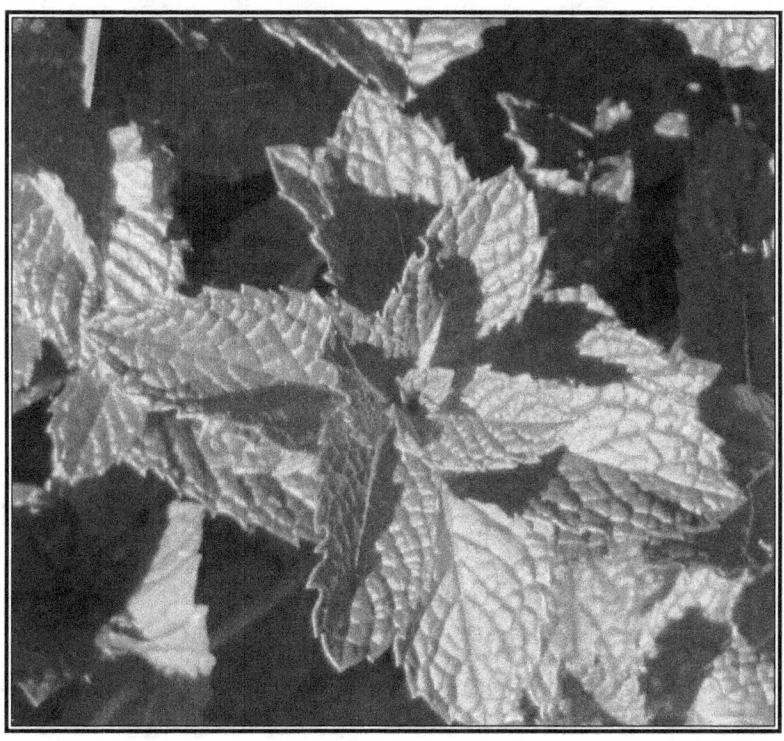

LEMON ESSENTIAL OIL

You can find many ways to use this versatile essential oil. It is useful for cooking and cleaning. Use it to uplift your mood and energize your body and mind while creating a healthy, fresh atmosphere in your home.

Take a deep breath of its fresh citrus scent to invigorate your mind and feel more mentally clear. *(Inhalation)*

Lemon essential oil is an excellent source of d-limonene. When taken internally it can help boost the immune system and help to fight off viruses and heal cold sores. *(Ingest)*

Rub a few drops on your the palms of your hands before going into a crowded space to deter germs. *(Topically)*

Lemon essential oil's strong citrus scent is energizing and uplifting. Its fresh citrus scent will invigorate your mind, body and spirit--INSTANTLY!

If you experience days filled with stress; or the world seems to be moving way too fast making you feel like a bunch of frazzled nerves, anxious or shaky, lemon essential oil may be just the ticket to uplift your spirits and calm your nerves. Use aromatherapy and diffuse lemon essential oil into your room to help relax your spirit. Diffuse or deeply breathe in lemon essential oil to spark a memory of playing on a sunny tropical beach to uplift your mood.

Dilute about 15 drops in a small spray bottle to help rid a home of strong food or pet odors. Spraying or diffusing lemon essential oil in the kitchen, or anywhere in your home or workplace can help to promote a feeling of freshness and crispness. It is much healthier for you and your family to breathe than commercially sold air fresheners.

Anxiety can cause insomnia for many people, which increases their feeling of being overly stressed. Try using lemon essential oil the next night when you just can't fall sleep. Diffuse it to help dispel worries and relieve anxious thoughts, without stimulating your brain to wakefulness. Or you can put a few drops on your palms, rub them together, place them over your nose and deeply breath it in. This can help you to sleep at night and feel less anxious during the day.

Lemon essential oil is very helpful if you are searching for a natural way to clean your home or workplace. Use lemon essential oil to spot clean everything from household surfaces to skin.

Apply lemon essential oil to quickly remove grease from kitchen surfaces. Put a drop on a dry paper towel and rub it on any greasy surface. Wait a moment, then rub it off with another paper towel or wet sponge. Put a few drops in hot water or on a sponge when cleaning greasy dishes and watch the grease fall away.

Create you own natural scouring powder. Fill a container with baking soda. Create a well in the center and add 15 or more drops of lemon oil into the well. Put the lid on the container and shake the solution. You can use it in your kitchen and bath areas for a great smelling, gentle on the hands cleansing powder that cuts grease and doesn't scratch surfaces.

Lemon essential oil can also be used as a disinfectant. Put a few drops on a wet cloth to clean kitchen and bathroom surfaces to discourage germs and create a very clean and fresh smelling in these rooms.

Mix baking soda and lemon essential oil together to create a natural carpet freshener. Sprinkle it around on the carpet, let it sit for a few minutes and then vacuum.

Lemon essential oil brakes down petrochemical products and is safer to use than gasoline or paint thinner. Sticky tar or gum comes off hands easily when lemon essential oil is applied directly to the area where it is stuck. Use it to remove labels without leaving behind a gummy residue.

Diffuse lemon essential oil in your space to help combat feelings of depression. Invite in a little drop of Nature to brighten your spirit and help chase the blues away. Take a few moments to breathe in this safe and natural cure for depression and sadness.

Use it to add some zest to your recipes. Add food grade lemon essential oil to foods like vinaigrettes and sorbets for additional flavor and gentle internal cleansing.

CREATE HEALTHY HOT OR COLD BEVERAGES

There are many food grade essential oils that can be used to create healthy soothing hot teas or refreshing cool beverages. Use a food grade quality of any of these three essential oils to create and enjoy a variety of healthy hot teas or cold drinks.

As an added benefit, you can use aromatherapy with these beverages. Add a few drops to a glass of cold water or a cup of hot water and slowly sip it. Breathe in the aroma. Allow yourself to enjoy the soothing aroma as it begins to relax your mind and spirit. Some oils will help you find a sense of serenity and transport yourself to a happier, more peaceful and relaxed space; others will help energize and uplift your spirit.

COLD DRINKS

Many people use caffeine and sugar filled drinks to get energized during the day. This is **NOT** a very healthy approach for getting energized. Instead, try adding a drop or two of peppermint essential oil to a glass of cold water. This makes a very refreshing and energizing cold drink. Take a drink and breathe in its energizing scent. You will quickly feel your mind and body feeling revitalized. This is a great way to naturally re-energize yourself any time of day.

When a person is happier and feeling less stressed, it is easier to work on weight management. Add a few drops of lavender, lemon or peppermint essential oil to a cold glass of purified or sparkling water to help relieve the desire for sugary or diet drinks and keep your mood uplifted at the same time. Add a drop of one of these food grade essential oils to a glass of water to help you lose a bit of weight by entertaining your taste buds and avoid the desire of grabbing a sugary or diet drink. Use them to make a drink with a very refreshing taste to help cut down cravings for sugar while giving you extra energy.

Lemon essential oil is perfect to add to pure water to create a refreshing and immune boosting drink while traveling or when you are among a large group of strangers anywhere.

Adding peppermint essential oil to a glass of water will help clear your sinuses and boost your immune system.

Hot Teas:

Try adding a few drops of food grade lavender, peppermint or lemon essential oil to your favorite tea instead of sugar to create a health giving and energizing drink and warm you on a cold day.

Adding a small amount of lavender essential oil to a cup of hot water creates a soothing tea to help settle your nerves any time of day. The benefit of its aroma wafting up from the cup helps speed its soothing energy throughout your mind.

Peppermint essential oil tea can also be a wonderful soothing tea. It has the added benefit of helping to cleanse and strengthen the entire body.

Nature has many herbs that can help relieve an upset stomach without creating another unnatural side effect that can sometimes be caused by using pharmaceutical products.

When you experience an upset or queasy stomach after you have eaten a new food or too much heavy foods at a party, adding a bit of an essential oil to a hot or cold drink can help give you instant, natural relief. You can use pure, food grade peppermint essential oil to create a soothing tea to aid with digestion or relieve stomach gas when experiencing indigestion. Put a drop or two in a cup of hot water for a soothing tea that internally helps relieve minor digestive discomfort.

Lavender essential oil tea can also be used to help relax the stomach muscles and relieve stomach gas. Lavender's soothing aroma will help you relax mentally, which will also aid digestion, as stress often prevents the digestive process from functioning properly. Breathe in the warm vapors of the tea to help relieve a headache which might accompany stomach discomfort caused by a bit too much party activity.

Create a soothing lavender essential oil tea to help you fall asleep at night and wake up feeling refreshed and energized in the morning.

OTHER BENEFITS

All three of these essential oils are helpful when dealing with colds, the flu or any type of congestion.

Peppermint essential oil tea works best to relieve congestion when suffering from a cold or the flu. This tea will help you find relief from a cold by reducing congested sinuses. Deeply inhale its gentle aroma to help break up the congestion in your lungs and stuffed up nose.

You can also use peppermint or lemon essential oil to create a tea to soothe a sore throat.

A cup of peppermint essential oil tea also offers headache relief. It helps strengthen the nerves instead of weakening them as aspirin and other drugs tend to do when used to relieve, inflammation, muscle pain or headaches. And, it is much easier on the stomach. Lavender essential oil tea is another headache relief aid. It relaxes the muscles and helps you find relief naturally.

IMPORTANT REMINDERS

Always use only 100% pure, food grade essential oils when ingesting them to avoid creating an unwanted health challenge that could come from lesser quality oils.

Always test your sensitivity to essential oils before ingesting them, even in small amounts.

Always use purified water or unadulterated sparkling water for drinking when you ingest food grade essential oils.

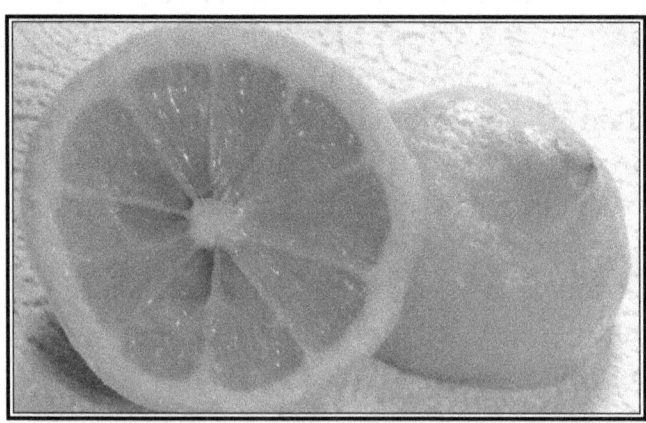

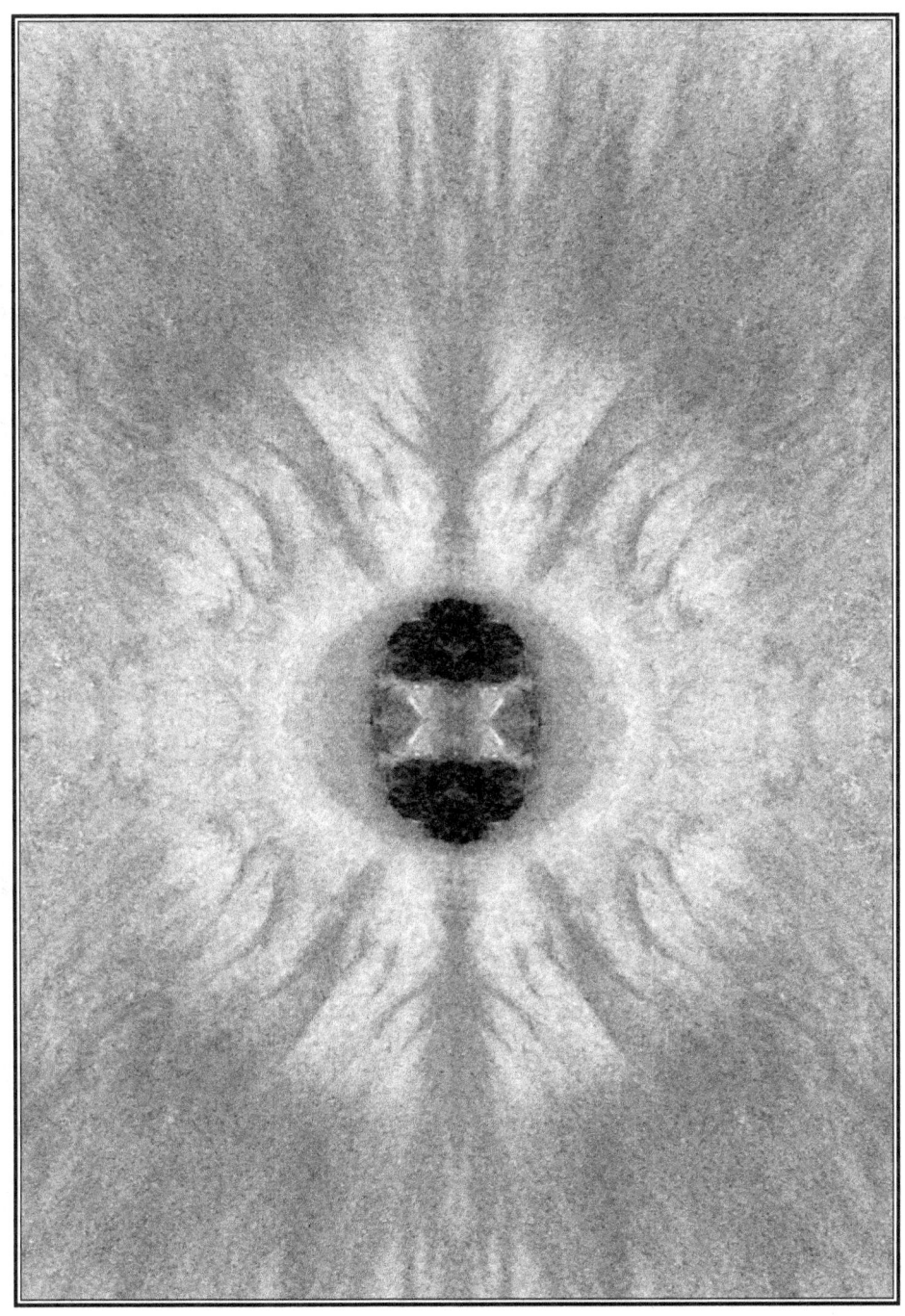

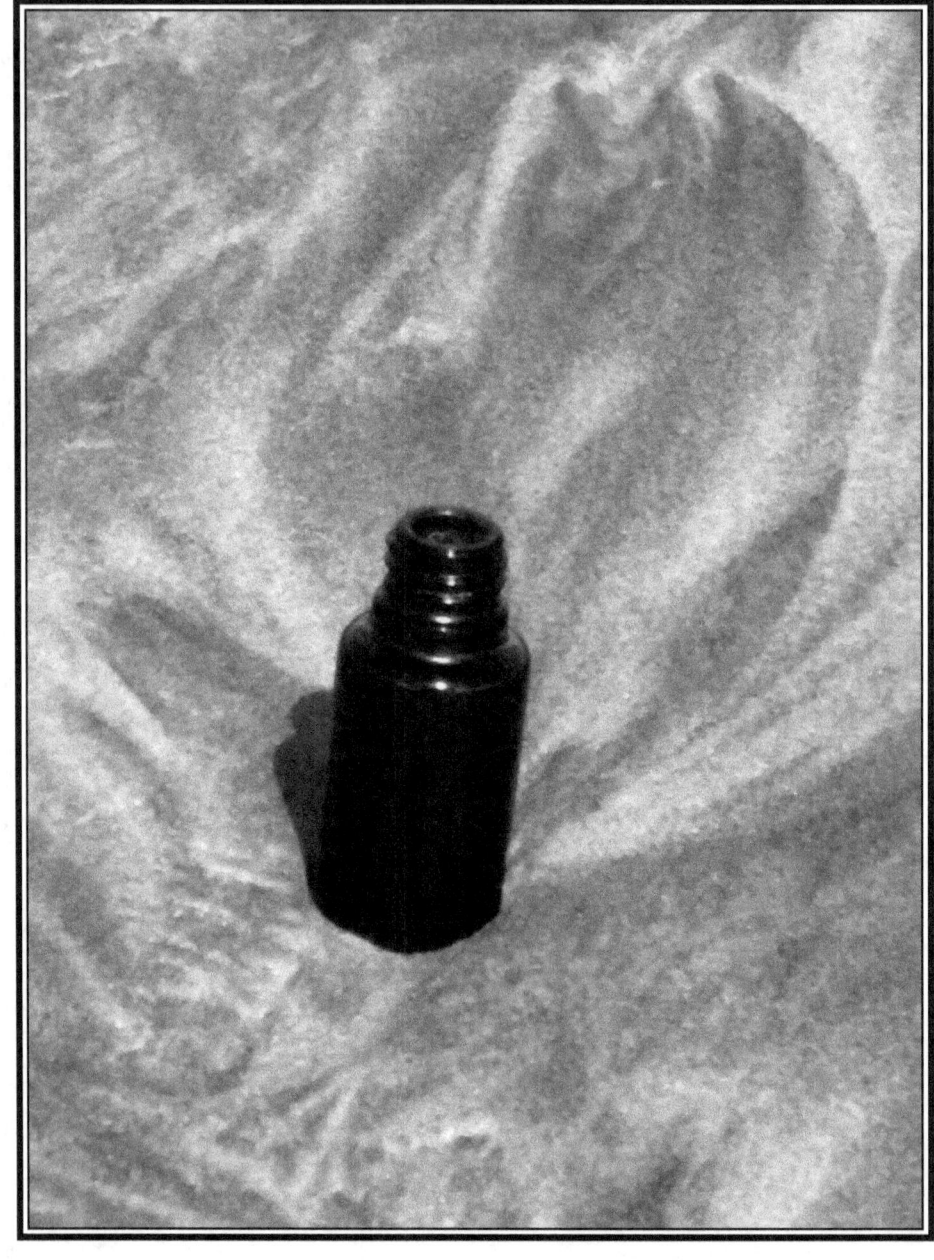

"TIPS" FOR USING ESSENTIAL OILS DISCLAIMER

Essential oils have been used in many cultures around the world for culinary and medicinal purposes for centuries. Nature's gifts have been distilled by people since almost the beginning of time.

On the following pages the properties of many essential oils will be defined and descriptions of ways you can try using them in your home or at work to make natural and safe changes to your health and life.

Most of these essential oils have a description of its scent.

All essential oils listed here have notes about how they have been used as a natural herbal remedy throughout history and currently.

Disclaimer

This information has been gathered from many reference sources and testimonials.

Just as all prescribed medications do not work for everyone in the same way, essential oils tend to work differently for every individual who uses them.

Many essential oils have the same healing properties as another. Some will work for one person, other essential oils for another person. Some work very quickly for one person, and not so quickly for another person. Test them for yourself to discover which essential oils work best for your particular health challenge.

Few essential oils have been tested in scientific studies and they are not regulated by the FDA.

Always remember that every BODY is different.

Everyone's constitution and bodies are different and react differently to everything they come into contact with, externally and internally. Your body knows what works.

Some people have allergies or negative reactions to different plants or a certain plant family. They may experience a negative reaction to an essential oil based on a specific plant, but they can use all the other essential oils.

Tolerances for amounts vary according to weight and age of each individual, especially when ingesting an oil.

Some people have very sensitive skin and need all oils to be applied in a natural carrier oil, others can tolerate direct application of every oil to their skin.

If you experience a burning sensation when you apply an essential oil full strength, apply a bit of olive oil and that should calm it down quickly.

Occasionally people experience skin irritation when using any essential oil full strength, whereas many people can use all essential oils full strength and experience positive healthy results.

Some people can ingest food-grade essential oils and receive a healing benefit without experiencing any negative reaction, other people may experience nausea usually due to the body detoxifying from the cleansing action of the oils.

This is usually a temporary and often beneficial effect.

Always TEST! any new essential oil in a very small amount before you consider using it in a larger amount.

About the *"Tips"*

These *"Tips"* are being passed on to you from the author, and friends of the author.

These essential oils *"Tips"* are based on how each one has worked for many people.

So some of these *"Tips"* will work for you, and others may not have the same effect for you as described in the notes. Every body reacts differently to everything it comes into contact with on a daily basis.

Everyone understands that some medications work for some people, whereas others may cause health problems or have unwanted side-effects, others just do nothing.

Essential oils very rarely cause any type of side-effect. If one does occur, it is most likely an allergic reaction to the plant itself and will not last long once you have washed off the oil or quit diffusing it in your room.

With this slight possibility in mind, it is suggested you always do a one drop test when trying a new essential oil on your body or in a drink or cooking with it.

Before massaging a new essential oil on a large area of your body, always test it on a small patch of your skin

Before ingesting any essential oil, always try a single drop of it. Always mix essential oils with Rice Milk, olive oil or water when taking them orally.

You will want to be careful when applying essential oils on the face or neck areas to avoid getting the oils or aromas to close to your eyes or in the inner ear.

It would be best to close your eyes and rest for a few moments after applying essential oils to the temples or forehead to avoid any possibility of irritating your eyes.

If an oil, such as peppermint, does get in the eye, the discomfort will probably be gone within a few short minutes. If needed, rinse with a pure vegetable oil *(do not use water to rinse out eye.)* Young Living Essential Oils therapeutic-grade oils will not damage the eye but can cause a pretty high degree of discomfort.

Cautions

Be sure to read the "Cautions" after the information sections.

Many essential oils are cleansing to the systems of the body and it is possible that using them could cause a *"cleansing or healing crisis"* by releasing toxins. In that case, stop or cut back on using the essential oil until symptoms subside, then very slowly introduce it again, allowing a gentler cleansing.

There are many types of essential oils, and they come from all over the World and from many different distributors.

All of the *"Tips"* in this book are based on using 100% therapeutic or food grade essential oils.

Of course, I have my favorite essential oils distributor as mentioned in a previous chapter. Still, I would recommend you do your own research to determine which essential oils will work best for your personal needs.

Please consider visiting my essential oils web page to learn more about Young Living Essential Oils and why that company is my first choice for where to purchase essential oils of high quality and proven results.

Visit my web site:http://www.youngliving.com/juliaw

Or if this book was shared with you by a friend, ask them to help you learn more about essential oils.

If you have lost contact with that person you might find their contact information at:

www.usingessentialoilsforhealth.com.

Please take a moment to read the below information section before reading further.

The following disclaimer applies to ALL of the Descriptions and *"Tips"* you find after many of the essential oil informative sections.

The following *"Tips"* are meant to give you suggestions about how to use essential oils in your every day life, including when giving or receiving massages; diffusing; aromatherapy; cooking; enjoying cold drinks or teas; or cleaning your home or workspace.

These "Tips" are not intended to diagnose, prevent, treat, or cure any disease."

The author assumes no liability for any damage caused by use of any of these essential oils "Tips".

The statements made in this book have not been evaluated by the Food and Drug Administration.

The FDA governs drugs, not nutraceuticals.

*FDA prioritizes reviewing and screening major food and drugs entering the market and rarely analyzes the safety and efficacy of any supplement. So **no** non-drug, herbal, natural health aids are FDA approved.*

Modern science has not validated many of the historical claims, but some have been researched by scientific tests with very positive and hopeful results for creating natural approaches to helping people gain their Optimum Health.

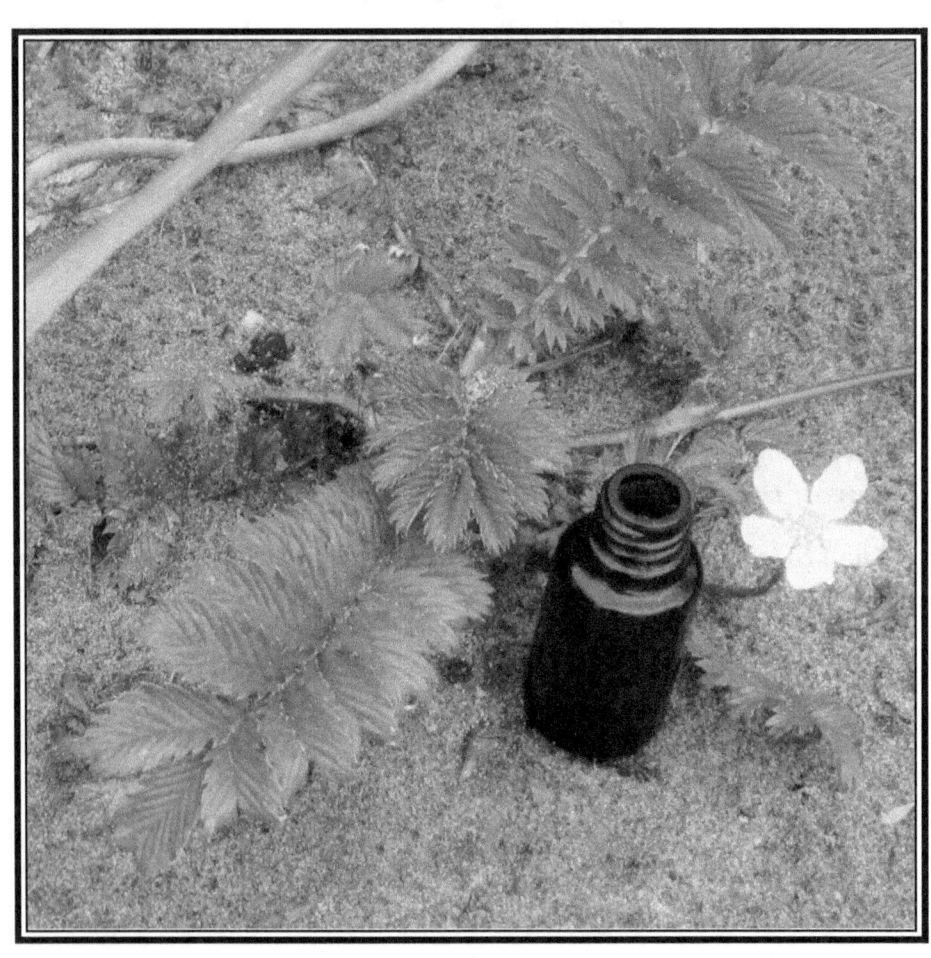

DESCRIPTIONS, HISTORICAL BACKGROUNDS AND "TIPS" FOR USING SINGLE ESSENTIAL OILS

On the following pages you will find descriptions of various essential oils that include a comment on their scent and some historical background.

This is by no means a complete list of all essential oils that exist, but includes the most popular and commonly used essential oils found all around the world.

Some are followed with *"Tips"*.

These *"Tips"* are suggested ways to use the therapeutic-grade essential oils that have been tested by myself or friends who have shared their successes using the essential oils.

Some have a *"Caution"* after the description.

Please pay careful attention to these.

Although most therapeutic or food grade essential oils are safe for use by everyone, certain ones are very strong or may have an adverse affect relating to pregnancy or certain health conditions.

Reminders:

Every body is different.

Not all essential oils work for everyone the same way.

TEST! a small amount of any new essential oil before using it in larger amounts.

Balsam Fir Oil is an uplifting scent. It can be useful to relieve many physical ailments.

Massage this essential oil when your body is feeling stiff to relax and soothe tight muscles.

Use it to relieve body discomfort associated with excessive exercise or when you didn't stretch well before.

It can be inhaled to help balance moods by promoting a sense of well-being and help to "ground" you.

Similar to frankincense, it helps to increase spirituality. It can be diffused when meditating to help go deeper within.

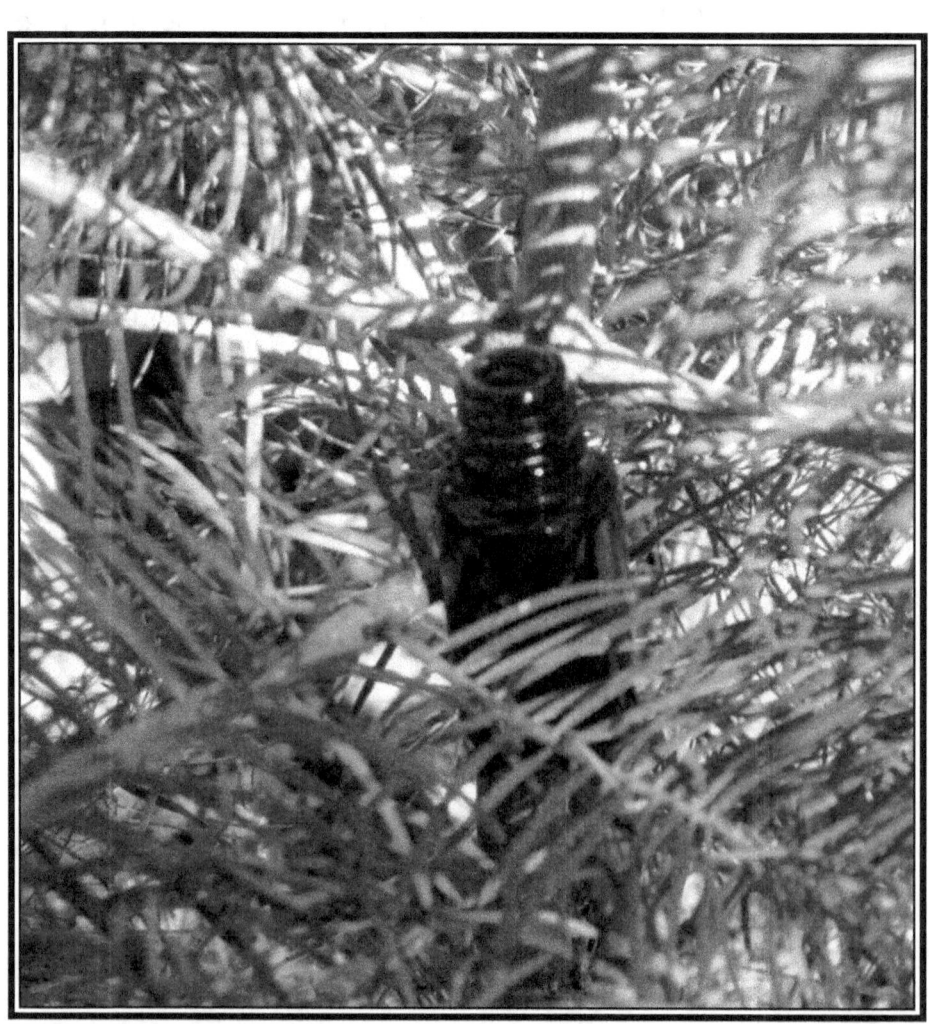

Basil Oil has a strong spicy aroma. Inhale it during times of fatigue to help you restore mental alertness and clarity. Take a deep breath in and it will refresh your mind.
When inhaled, it may sharpen your sense of smell.
When applied topically, it can relax tense, tired and sore muscles.

Tip: Add zest to steamed vegetables. Put a drop or two of basil, rosemary or thyme essential oils in the water you are using to steam the vegetables.
Tip: When cooking an Italian meal, add a few drops of basil essential oil for healthy, authentic flavoring.

----------- ----------- ---------- ---------- ----------- ----------- ------------ ----------- ---------

Bergamot Oil has a light citrus aroma. Historically it was used in the Middle East to help oily complexions. It is used in Earl Grey Tea to give it a distinct flavor.
It has about 300 chemical constituents that contribute to its refreshing mood-lifting qualities.
When inhaled, it may help to build confidence and uplift your mind and spirit out of a depressed mood.
Women find it very helpful during their monthly cycles.

Caution: Bergamot essential oil is very photosensitive and should NOT be applied to the skin that will be exposed to direct sunlight or ultra-violet light within 12 hours.

Tip: Diffuse bergamot oil during times of stress to help relax and become more focused on the task at hand.

----------- ----------- ---------- ---------- ----------- ----------- ------------ ----------- ---------

Cedarwood Oil has a woody, balsamic, warm aroma.
This essential oil contains the constituent cedrol which is known to help promote relaxation, balance and increase mental focus.
When used as a dietary supplement or inhaled, it can help maintain healthy lung function.
It has a relaxing and soothing effect when used for massage.

Tip: Diffuse this oil and lets its aroma take your mind on a journey into a beautiful pine forest and help forget the cares of the day.

----------- ----------- ---------- ---------- ----------- ----------- ------------ ----------- ---------

Chamomile Oil is best known for its calming and relaxing properties. It has a gentle flowery scent.

There are two species of the plant: Roman and German. They belong to the same family as asters and daisies. Chamomile's powerful healing properties come from a complex blend of substances found in the flowering heads. When they are distilled, they yield an azure-blue volatile oil.

This is another extremely versatile essential oil.

Chamomile essential oil has anti-inflammatory, antispasmodic and analgesic properties.

This essential oil has been used to help with many health challenges including headaches, indigestion, and nervousness. It is helpful in relieving painful aching muscles and joints.

The herb has been used to relieve swelling from arthritis, sprains and in joints.

Herbalist also use it to help heal burns and relieve itchy skin.

This essential oil can be applied topically to calm down a queasy stomach.

It is used in many natural hair products.

Roman Chamomile is great for relieving itching. It may not heal the cause but the itching will stop.

Caution: Chamomile oil is considered one of the safest essential oils, but there is a chance of an allergic reaction for people who suffer from hay fever. If you are allergic to ragweed, chrysanthemums, or daisies, be cautious about drinking the tea, inhaling or applying it to your skin. TEST!

Tip: When used as a tea, chamomile can help quiet an upset stomach, quench the fires of inflammation and bring a restful night's sleep.

Tip: When suffering from a cold and the sniffles, add a few drops to a steaming pan of water, lean over it and inhale the steam. The stronger the aroma, the more effective it is.

Tip: Add drops of chamomile oil to warm water, let it cool and use it as a refreshing rinse for hair and body.

----------- ----------- ---------- ---------- ----------- ----------- ------------ ---------- ---------

Cinnamon Bark Oil comes from the bark of an Asian tree and has a long history for healing a variety of health challenges and used in variety of culinary dishes.

Ancient Chinese herbalists mention it as early as 2700 B.C. They recommended the herb for fever, diarrhea and menstrual problems.

In the Bible, Moses used it in holy anointing oil.

Egyptians used it as an ingredient in embalming mixtures for their mummies.

The twelfth-century German herbalist Hildegard from Bingen recommended it as *"the universal spice for sinuses."* and to treat colds, flu, and cancer.

It is believed to have antiseptic properties and is supportive of the body's natural defenses.

It also helps sooth the stomach which in turn may help prevent ulcers.

Cinnamon is found in many natural toothpastes. Its antiseptic property may help kill the bacteria that cause tooth decay and gum disease.

Caution: Cinnamon essential oil is very strong and should be used sparingly if taken internally.
TEST! your tolerance.

Caution: Don't use it for too many days in a row.

Caution: Always dilute this very potent essential oil in a pure vegetable carrier oil when applying topically. TEST!

Tip: Try adding a few drops of cinnamon bark essential oil to water boiling on the stove to create an inviting holiday atmosphere and add a warm and welcoming feeling to a wintery home.

Tip: Add a drop to apple cider or a cup of tea to spice it up.

Tip: Use a cup of cinnamon essential oil tea to sooth a troubled stomach.

Tip: When baking, add a drop or two to create more flavorful, spicy cakes and cookies to give a taste of the holidays all year long.

Citronella Oil is one of the essential oils obtained from the leaves and stems of different species of Cymbopogon. This oil is used in soap, perfumery, cosmetic and flavoring industries throughout the world. It can be used to sanitize and deodorize surfaces.

Citronella essential oil may help with colds, fatigue, flu, headaches, and neuralgia.

Research also shows that citronella oil has strong antifungal properties.

Combining it with cedarwood essential oil, it makes excellent insect repellent. It is also a renowned plant-based insect repellent, and has been registered for this use in the United States since 1948. The United States Environmental Protection Agency considers oil of citronella as a biopesticide with a non-toxic mode of action.

Tip: *Spray water with drops of this essential oil in it around outdoor eating areas to discourage bugs.*

Tip: *Diffuse it as a way to calm barking dogs.*

Tip: *Place cotton balls or a cloth with drops of citronella oil in closets or the bottom of plastic bags when storing wools, furs or feathery items to dissuade moths.*

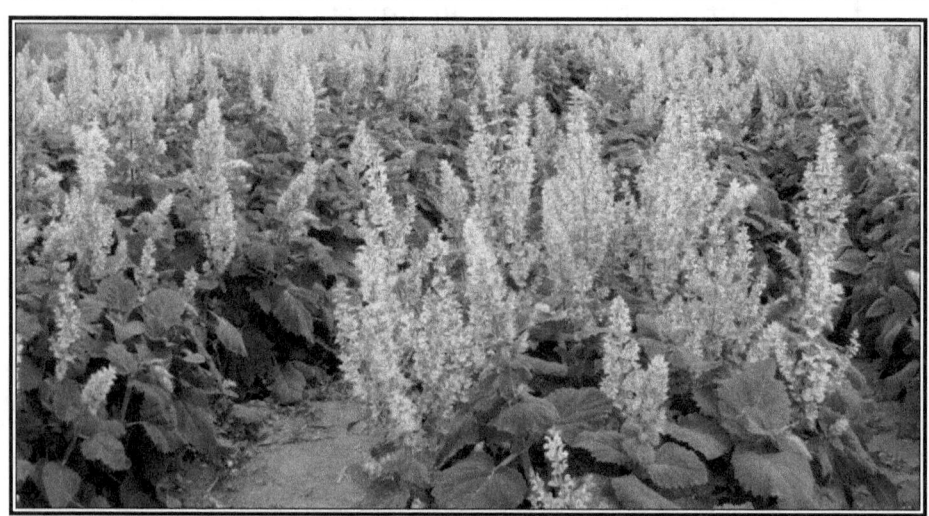

Clary Sage Oil has a herbaceous aroma that helps calm nerves. Its mellow, warm, herbal scent is uplifting and relaxing to the mind and body.

It contains natural pytoestrogens.

For women, it can help support a normal, healthy attitude during menopause and during PMS. Use it to ease menstrual discomfort. Diffuse it to relax the mind, relieve stress and balance moodiness.

When massaged into lower back and hips, it helps relieve pain and tight joints.

Diffuse it in the bedroom to enhance the ability to dream and as a natural way to help relax into a deep and restful sleep.

Clove Oil has a sweet, spicy scent that can be stimulating and revitalizing when inhaled after a long tiring day.

Clove is nature's strongest antioxidant. It has immune-enhancing properties as its principal constituent is eugenol, which is used in the dental industry. Eugenol makes the herb effective as an antiseptic and painkiller. It has been used for many years in home remedies to numb the gums and help kill bacteria and viruses.

Clove essential oil can be used to fight digestive disorders. Be sure you always dilute it in water, olive oil or rice milk before ingesting.

Poultices of clove essential oil can be used on the skin to promote healing of cuts and bites. Studies have shown it can kill several strains of staphylococcus bacteria and other organisms that can cause infection in the skin.

Caution: Always dilute clove essential oil in a pure vegetable carrier oil for topical use.

Caution: Be sure to dilute it in rice milk, olive oil or pure water before ingesting.

Tip: Try three drops of clove essential oil in a glass of water when constipated. Don't overdo.

Tip: *Pure, food-grade clove essential oil can be used in cooking and baking.*

Tip: *Try adding a few drops to water boiling on the stove to add a warm and welcoming feeling to a wintery home.*

Coriander Oil has a sweet, warming fragrance. It has been used for thousands of years for cooking and in medicinal natural remedies.

Coriander comes from the same plant as cilantro. Coriander is the name for the seeds and cilantro is the name for the leaves.

It can aid digestion and soothe an upset stomach when taken as a dietary supplement.

It is also believed to support pancreatic function and helps to strengthen the heart.

Coriander has antibacterial properties and can help prevent infections in wounds and insect bites.

Studies have suggested that it has anti-inflammatory properties and may help alleviate pain caused by arthritis.

Tip: *Use pure coriander essential oil to cook Indian curry style meals.*

Cypress Oil has a lightly evergreen herbaceous aroma.

Diffuse it to help restore feelings of security and stability.

It can be especially comforting during the winter season when we are unable to spend much time outdoors.

Cypress essential oil can help stimulate circulatory health when massaged onto the body.

Tip: *Apply a drop on a bruise once or twice a day. It usually disappears within days, rather than weeks.*

Tip: *Try massaging a bit of cypress essential oil in a carrier oil onto your feet and hands before going outside on a wintery day. Helps keep circulation flowing and body parts warmer.*

Dill Oil has been used throughout history for its culinary and medicinal properties.

Add a few drops to water to soothe the stomach and aid digestion. It can also be applied topically to the stomach area to relieve an upset stomach.

It is reputed to help prevent gas. The herb exhibits anti-foaming actions that may help break up gas bubbles forming in the stomach.

Dill essential oil has been show to support pancreatic function.

Apply it to the bottom of the feet to help calm a troubled mind.

Tip: Add a few drops to olive oil when creating a healthy, flavorful oil and vinegar salad dressing.

Elemi Oil originated in the Philipines and is in the same botanical family as frankincense and myrrh.

Europeans traditionally use it for skin tone and protection.

Add it to a carrier oil and massage it into sore or stressed muscles when you have overdone your exercise routine or taken a very long hike or run.

Similar to frankincense, it has antibacterial properties and can help in healing cuts or bug bites. In the 17th century, J. J. Wecker, a physician, applied it in an ointment to soldiers wounded on the battlefield to avoid infection.

Tip: Diffuse to help clear your mind and help deepen meditation.

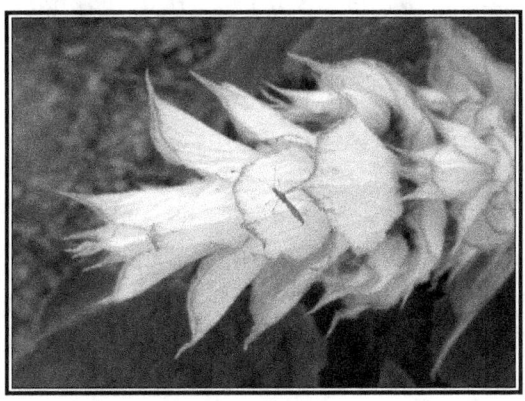

Eucalyptus Oil was discovered in Australia and different species create oils in a variety of strengths and have different uses.

All varieties have an invigorating, unique and refreshing aroma. It is an excellent oil to diffuse.

When treating colds and coughs, it loosens phlegm in the lungs.

Eucalyptus leaf essential oil contains a chemical, eucalyptol, that has decongestant and antiseptic qualities.

Eucalyptus essential oil also has been shown to kill several types of bacteria and viruses.

It is often used to support the respiratory system. It can help asthma suffers breathe easier also.

Some varieties are well suited to topical use to soothe muscles after exercise.

Eucalyptus essential oil diluted in a bit of pure vegetable oil can be applied to cuts and bites to help prevent infection.

Research has proven that when applied topically, it increases blood flow to muscle tissue, and helps relieve sore muscles.

Caution: Never ingest any eucalyptus essential oil!
     Be very aware that when ingested it can be highly poisonous, even fatal!

Tip: Mix baking soda and eucalyptus essential oil together to create a natural carpet freshener. Sprinkle it around on the carpet, let it sit for a minute or two and then vacuum.

Tip: When suffering from a cold and the sniffles, add a few drops to steaming pan of water, lean over it and inhale the steam. The stronger the aroma, the more effective it is.

Tip: Add a few drops to a bath when feeling under the weather or your muscles are achy.

----------- ----------- ---------- ---------- ----------- ----------- ------------ ----------- ---------

Eucalyptus Blue Oil is offered exclusively by Young Living.

It is high in the powerful constituent eucalyptol and promotes increased respiratory health. Diffuse it or rub it on the chest to relieve respiratory complaints that have interfered with enjoying your favorite activities.

It also can be used as an insect deterrent inside the home and out-of-doors.

Tip: Rub a few drops of eucalyptus blue in a carrier oil on your ankles, wrists and back of neck to discourage insects when engaged in outdoor activities.

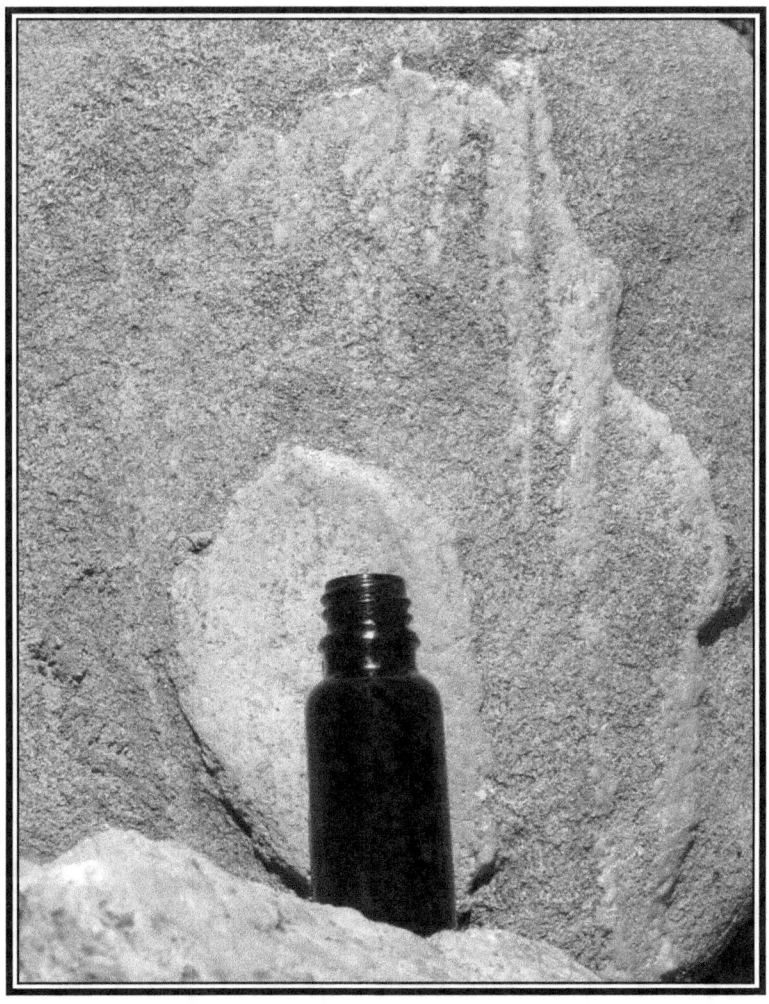

Frankincense Oil has a sweet, warm balsamic aroma.

In the Middle East, it has been considered a holy anointing oil and has been used for thousands of years in some cultures religious ceremonies.

Its aroma can stimulate and elevate the mind. Use it when trying to focus the mind.

Diffuse it in times of stress or despair to redirect your thoughts to a peaceful, joyful and more elevated place.

Frankincense's high frequency positively affects the immune and nervous systems, as well as bringing emotional balance.

It is also used in skin care products for dry and aging skin.

Tip: Diffuse to help clear your mind and deepen meditation.

Tip: For softer and smoother skin try rubbing frankincense on your face or stretch marks for a week.

Tip: Try using frankincense on small skin cancers. Rub it on the spots every morning and night for a week. Be sure to use a therapeutic-grade of this essential oil and consult with your doctor to oversee your progress.

Tip: During Cold and Flu Season, to keep germs at bay, rub frankincense essential oil under your nose before entering into places where you will be mingling with many people.

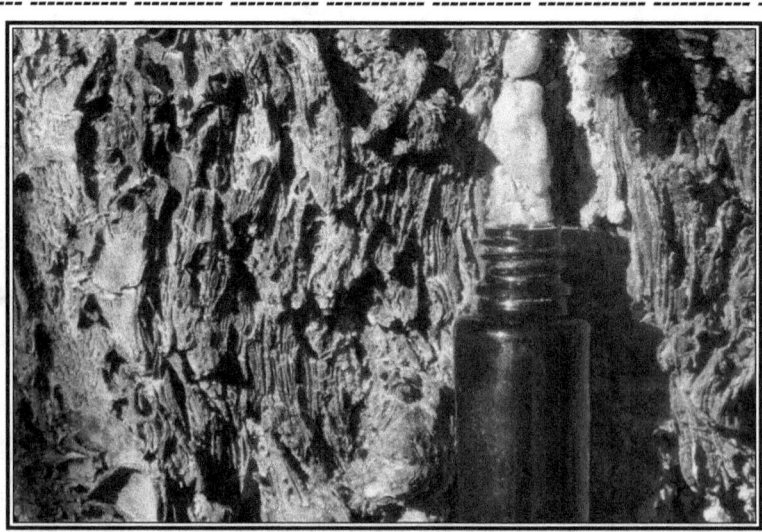

Geranium Oil has an uplifting, calming flowery scent.

Traditionally it is used to support the circulatory and nervous system. It helps to regulate the thyroid hormone and revitalize body tissue.

Geranium & rose essential oils have been found to have a gentle balancing effect on hormone levels. They also have the additional benefit of reducing stress.

Diffuse it to help release negative memories or thoughts.

It is especially beneficial to massage it over the liver and stomach area, the lower ribs and upper abdomen.

Use it as you would a deodorant and apply it in the under arms area.

It is excellent for the skin.

Tip: Try a few drops of geranium essential oil in your bath water or apply it directly on your skin to help lift fatigue.

Ginger Oil comes from what looks like a root, but botanically is a rhizome, or underground stem.

It has a spicy fragrance that is very energizing.

It is often used to support the digestive system to relieve indigestion and gas.

It can help reduce the feeling of nausea relating to motion sickness and the flu.

Ginger essential oil appears to work directly on the stomach as well as on the brain to calm the feeling of nausea.

It may help relieve arthritic knee pain and rheumatoid arthritis symptoms.

Ginger is antimicrobial.

Ginger can be found in many oral health products.

Various reports have linked the use of ginger to headache relief, lowering of blood cholesterol, relief from gout and prevention of stomach ulcers.

Ginger essential oil is useful in food preparation for a spicy addition to many recipes that is also very healthy.

Tip: *Try adding a couple of drops of ginger essential oil to a cup of tea to sooth a troubled stomach.*

Tip: *When preparing a stir-fry meal and you don't have fresh ginger root, add a few drops of ginger essential oil at the end of the cooking time for a healthy flavorful addition to the dish.*

Grapefruit Oil has a citrus, zesty sweet scent that is very uplifting and revitalizing for the spirit and emotions.

It is a very powerful antioxidant. A couple drops in water helps enhance your immune system. Similar to lemon essential oil, it contains the cell protectant d-limonene.

Grapefruit essential oil's fresh citrus aroma can energize and uplift your spirits. Diffuse it to change your mind-set when feeling stressed or sad.

It is nourishing to the skin and is a popular oil used in conjunction with weight management.

Use it to enhance the flavor of foods and water.

Caution: *Do not apply grapefruit essential oil to skin that will be exposed to direct sun or ultraviolet light within 12 hours.*

Caution: *As with after consuming most citrus fruits and oils, it is suggested that you don't brush your teeth for at least 30 minutes after ingesting to protect the tooth enamel.*

Tip: *To help with weight loss, add a few drops to a cold glass of plain or sparkling water to enjoy an energizing and refreshing drink and help relieve cravings for sugary or diet drinks.*

Helichrysum Oil is known for providing excellent support to the skin, liver, circulatory and nervous system.

It is also known for its restorative properties.

Helichrysum essential oil also provides a defense against harmful free radicals.

It supports healthy nerves and can be helpful for increasing circulation in your body.

Historically, it has been used to minimize bruising and ease varicose veins.

Applied topically helichrysum essential oil may help to clear skin blemishes and bruises.

Hyssop Oil has a slightly sweet scent.

It is a member of the mint family. Mint plants produce a volatile oil that gives them their distinct flavors. A chemical in these volatile oils helps to relieve irritations of the respiratory tract and nasal congestion.

This oil was considered a sacred oil and used in ceremonies by ancient Egyptians and Greeks.

In Biblical times it was used for its purifying properties.

Historically, it was used for healing respiratory problems such as bronchitis, coughs, hoarseness, sore throats and colds.

It has shown antiviral qualities in some studies.

Hyssop essential oil helps to support all systems in the body.

Tip: Add a couple of drops to a cup of tea to break up congestion when experiencing a cold. Add honey or lemon to taste.

Jasmine Oil has an exotic floral fragrance.

It is purported to help enhance self-confidence.

Diffuse or inhale it to relax, soothe, and uplift your spirit.

This is a popular perfume fragrance and has been used for attracting romantic encounters throughout the ages.

It helps balance feminine energy in the body.

Tip: Diffuse jasmine essential oil when inviting someone to your home for a romantic dinner.

Tip: Add to your bath waters or Epsom salts for a relaxing and soothing bath for both body and spirit.

Juniper Oil is extracted from juniper berries and has an earthy, woody scent.

Ancient Egyptian doctors used it as a laxative, and over time has been used to treat numerous ailments.

This is a very potent oil and caution should be used when ingesting or applying to the skin.

It is a powerful diuretic and has been used internally for purification and cleansing, but use it sparingly.

When diffused, its scent can help to promote spirituality and encourage self-esteem.

When used topically, diluted in a pure vegetable oil, it can help with oily skin.

And yes, it is used to make Gin.

Caution: Because of juniper essential oil's powerful diuretic effect, it can be harmful to someone with kidney problems. Use extreme caution if you have any kidney disease or stones.

Caution: Under no circumstances should a pregnant women use juniper essential oil in any form.

----------- ----------- ---------- ---------- ----------- ---------- ------------ ----------- ---------

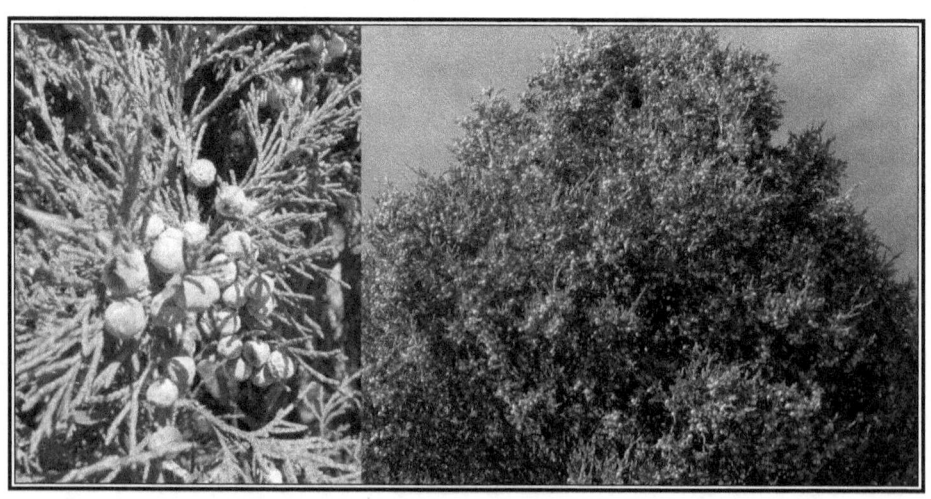

Lavender Oil has a herbaceous, sweet floral aroma that is both soothing and refreshing.

Lavender essential oil is one of the most versatile of all essential oils. No home should be without it.

It is an adaptogen and can assist the body when adapting to stress or imbalances. It aids winding down and relaxing before bedtime, yet can also boost stamina and energy during the day. It calms, uplifts, relaxes, rejuvenates, relieves, comforts and revives both the mind and body.

Lavender is highly regarded for healthy skin. It can be found in many natural skin and hair care products.

Use it to help cleanse cuts, bruises, and skin irritations. It fights germs on skin and in the air.

Lavender has balancing properties that when inhaled or massaged on the body can help relieve extreme stress.

Diffuse it in the bedroom in the evening to aid one to fall asleep quickly and get a good night's rest.

Placing some drops on a cloth or a few cotton balls in closets can help to keep moths from damaging fur, feathers and clothing.

Lavender imparts a delicate flavor when cooking with it. Lavender honey is a delightful addition to baking and teas.

Tip: Inhale lavender essential oil to relax your mind when entering or leaving a stressful situation.

Tip: If you have the hiccups, put a couple of drops of lavender essential oil in your hands. Rub them across your upper abdomen and your diaphragm to find relief quickly.

Tip: Place a few drops of lavender essential oil on a cotton ball and place it under your pillow for a peaceful nights rest.

Tip: Put drops of lavender essential oil on a cloth. Place it in a small plastic zippered pouch. Bring it when your traveling. Open the pouch in front of your nose and breathe in its aroma about every 30 minutes.

Tip: Place a drop on your underarms to keep odor down.

Tip: Place a drop of lavender essential oil on the a cotton ball under your pillow for enhanced relaxation during sleep.

Tip: Mix baking soda and lavender oil together to create a carpet freshener. Sprinkle it around on the carpet, let it sit for a minute or two and then vacuum the house to add a fresh scent where every you go.

Tip: Lavender also helps to keep stored linens smelling fresh. Put a few drops on a cloth or cotton balls. Replace the cloth or cotton balls, or just add more drops every month for the best results.

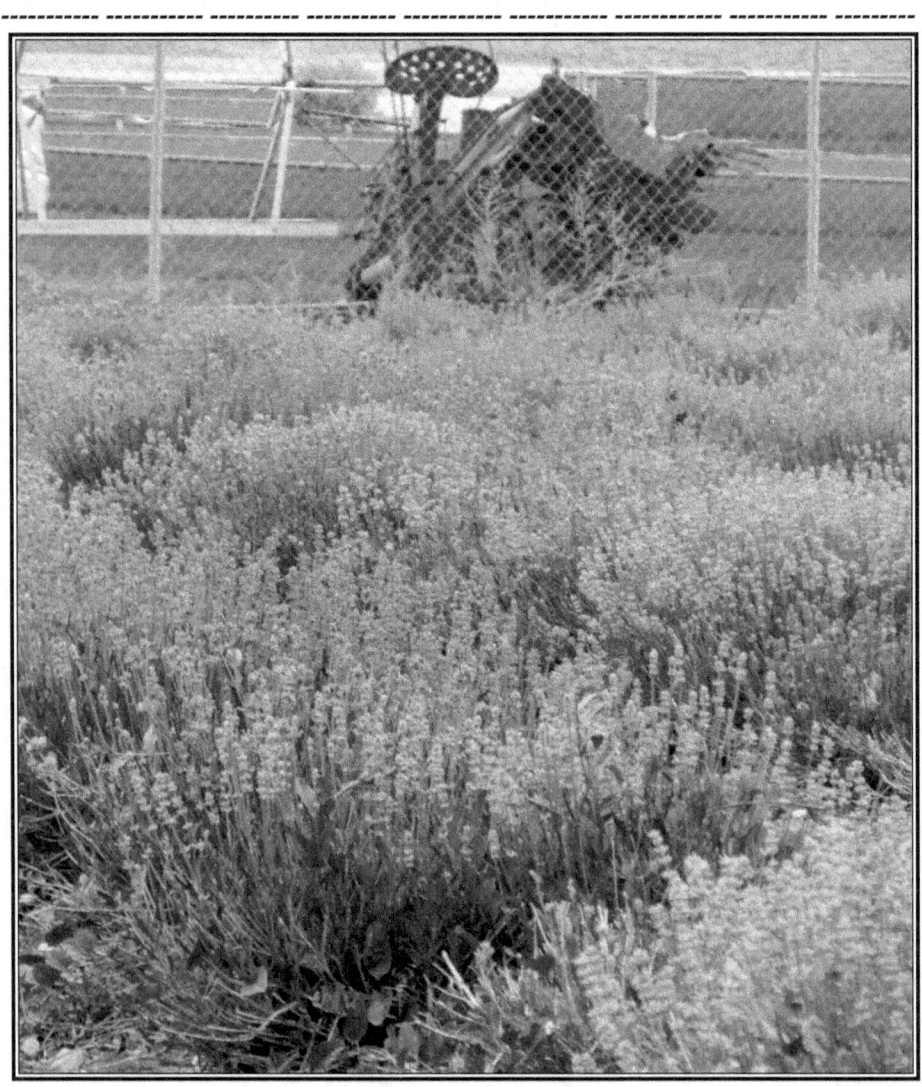

Lemon Oil has a fresh citrus scent that helps to invigorate the mind and promotes mental clarity. Its strong citrus scent is very revitalizing and uplifting.

You can find many ways to use this multipurpose essential oil, from cooking and cleaning to creating a fresh atmosphere in your home and that helps uplift your mood when inhaled.

Use it as a quick pick-me-up to regain energy during the day. Taken internally it can help boost the immune system as it is an excellent source of d-limonene.

To help stay on a diet, add a few drops to your plain or sparkling water or any natural beverage for a very refreshing taste that helps cut down cravings for sugar and easily replace unhealthy diet drinks.

Caution: As with after consuming most citrus fruits and oils, it is suggested you don't brush your teeth for at least 30 minutes after ingesting to protect tooth enamel.

Caution: DO NOT be apply citrus oils to skin that will be exposed to direct sunlight or ultra-violet light within 12 hours.

Tip: Add a touch of lemon essential oil when diffusing stronger-smelling oils.

Tip: Put lemon essential oil on a tissue or diffuse for a boost to the emotions, or the help promote mental clarity.

Tip: Place a drop of lemon essential oil on the a cotton ball under your pillow for enhanced relaxation during sleep.

Tip: Use it to spot clean everything from household surfaces to your skin.

Tip: Use it for cleaning greasy dishes and removing labels. A drop on a dry paper towel works best when trying to remove the residue from a label or grease on cabinets. Rub it on, wait a moment, then rub it off with a wet sponge.

Tip: Mix baking soda and lemon essential oil together to create a natural carpet freshener. Sprinkle it around on the carpet, let it sit for a minute or two and then vacuum.

Tip: Lemon essential oil makes a great air deodorizer and freshener. Add five drops of lemon essential oil and two drops of peppermint essential oil to one cup of pure water. Shake and spray for a fresh smelling home.

Tip: It can safely be used to remove tar or grease from hands and skin. Lemon essential oil brakes down petrochemical products and is safer to use than gasoline or paint thinner.

Tip: Fill a container with a small box of baking soda. Create a well in the center and pour thirty drops or more of lemon essential oil. Put the lid on the container and shake the solution. This is a great cleansing powder for the kitchen and bath that smells great, is gentle on the hands, cuts grease and doesn't scratch surfaces.

Tip: Try rubbing stains on dentures with lemon essential oil before soaking in denture cleaner.

Tip: Use it to add some lemony zest to your recipes.

Tip: Add lemon essential oil to foods like vinaigrettes and sorbets for additional flavor and gentle internal cleansing.

Tip: Massage lemon essential oil into cellulitis to help improve circulation and eliminate waste from the cells.

Tip: Add 10-15 drops of lemon essential oil to a gallon of carpet cleaning solutions to help pull out stains, brighten carpets, and leave a fresh smell in the room.

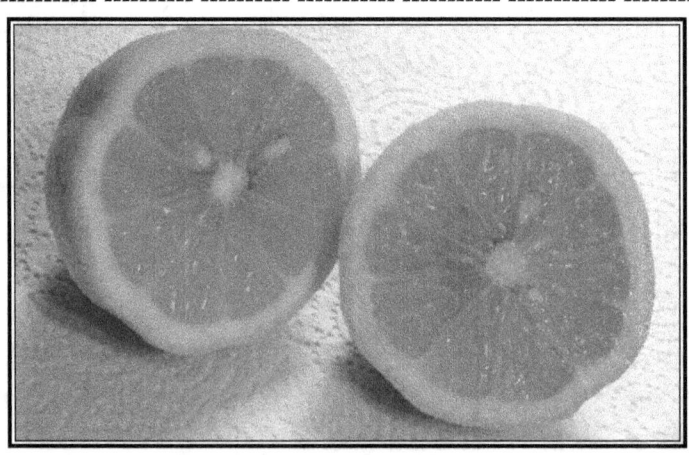

Lemongrass Oil has earthy undertones one detects along with its light citrus aroma.

Lemongrass helps support the circulatory system.

It inspires positive thoughts and helps to improve mental clarity.

Diffuse it to help refresh and rejuvenate the spirit. Use it to help bring back balance into your life.

Traditionally it has been used as a digestive aid. More recently it is applied topically and scores high on the antioxidant scale.

Lemongrass essential oil can help to regenerate ligaments and connective tissue.

Massage it onto sore or tired feet to get the spring back into your step.

Tip: *Spray lemongrass essential oil on linens to keep spiders or other unfriendly bugs from crawling into bed with you or your children.*

Marjoram Oil has a spicy scent. Historically it has been used for its culinary and medicinal properties in many cultures.

Considered a good tonic for overall health and can help improve a person's appetite.

As with many culinary uses, it can help relieve a sour stomach or indigestion.

It has a slight diuretic property and may help increase urine flow.

It is useful for relieving the pain caused by toothaches or headaches.

Traditionally, marjoram essential oil was used to ease muscle spasms. Massage marjoram essential oil into any sore or tense muscles for quick relief.

Diffuse it in your room or massage onto your temples and the back of the neck to help relieve nervous tension.

Marjoram essential oil can give relief from itchy insect bites and its antiseptic properties help prevent infection.

Tip: *When cooking an Italian meal, add some marjoram essential oil for healthy, authentic flavoring.*

Melaleuca Oil has high levels of terpineol and is highly regarded for its antibacterial properties.

Melaleuca essential oil can be very supportive of the body's immune system and natural defenses.

Historically, it has been used to ease a wide range of ailments and prevent infection.

It is found in many skin care products.

Young Living Essential Oils has five varieties of melaleuca oil.

Melaleuca Alternifolia is commonly know as Tea Tree Oil and used for treating fungal infections.

It has been used to treat candida, ringworm, sinus and lung infections, tooth and gum disease, water retention, hypertension, and skin conditions, such as acne, sores.

Tip: After cleaning a wound or bug bite, apply it topically to help prevent infection and aid quick healing.

Melissa Oil has a unique lemony, grassy aroma.

It is know for its purifying and cleansing properties.

Historically, it has been used to help balance emotions. The aroma from this gentle and delicate plant helps to bring out those characteristics in a person.

Several studies have shown it to be very beneficial when applied to the skin.

Melissa essential oil is used for viral infections (herpes, etc.), depression, anxiety, and insomnia.

Young Living cultivates this amazing plant in the fertile ground and cool, damp weather conditions found in St. Maries, Idaho. Each plant yields a very small amount of oil and YL has perfected the process of distilling the oil to create an all natural melissa essential oil.

Mountain Savory Oil has an invigorating scent.

It scores high on the antioxidant ORAC scale and its strong purifying properties supports the body's natural defenses and immune system.

Historically, it has been used as a general tonic for the body. It has been used to energize, invigorate and stimulate the body towards better health.

----------- ----------- ---------- ---------- ----------- ----------- ------------ ----------- ---------

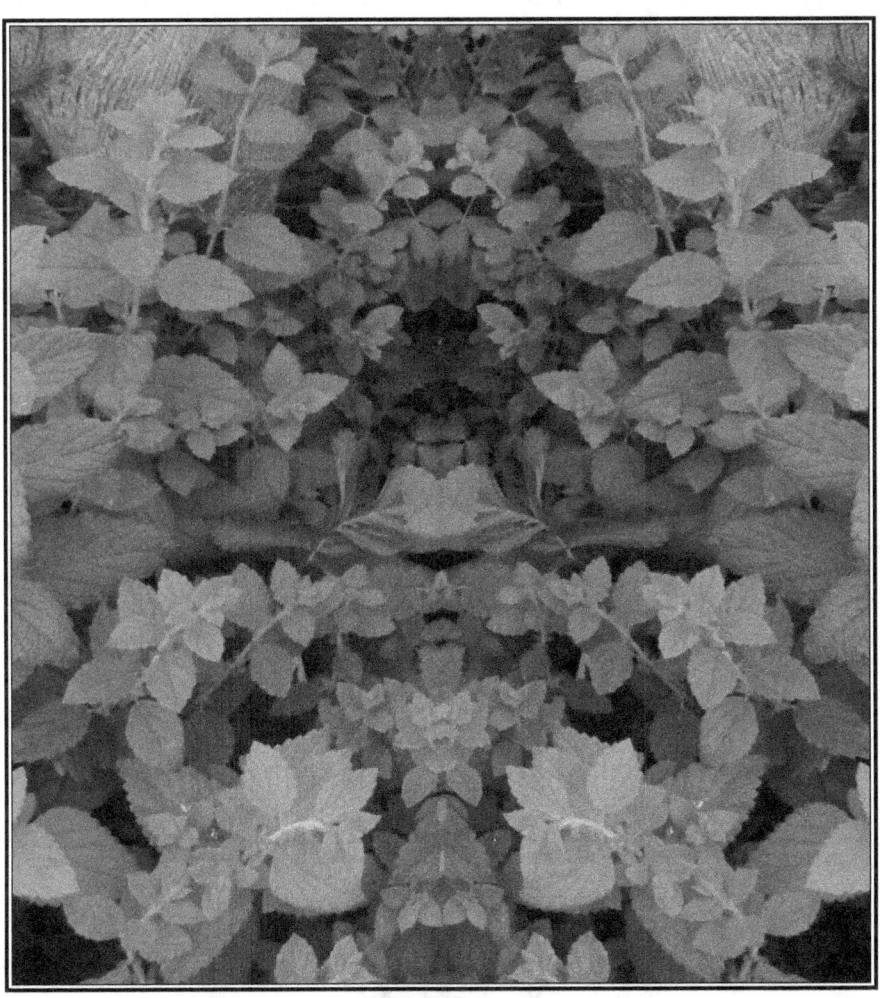

Myrrh Oil is an ancient Bible remedy that is still used today.

It has one of the highest levels of sesquiterpenes, a class of compounds that have direct effects on the hypothalamus, pituitary gland and amygdala, the seat of all our emotions.

Diffuse it to help reset your mind-set from stressed to relaxed; from sad to happy; or nervous to relaxed.

Myrrh essential oil has antiseptic properties that make it very useful for healing.

Diffuse it to stimulate deeper breathing and loosen phlegm in the chest to aid in finding relief for bronchial and all chest and lung diseases.

It is very supportive of the body's natural cellular repair process. Use it for bathing any sores on the body. Add a few drops to a pure carrier oil and apply topically to dry, chapped, cracked or wrinkled skin and feel the difference in just a few days.

Myrrh essential oil is commonly found in commercial oral hygiene products. Add a few drops to a small amount of water and use as a gargle to help keep gums healthy, heal mouth sores, and removes bad breath.

Tip: Diffuse Myrrh essential oil when preparing to do meditation for a deeper, more spiritual experience.

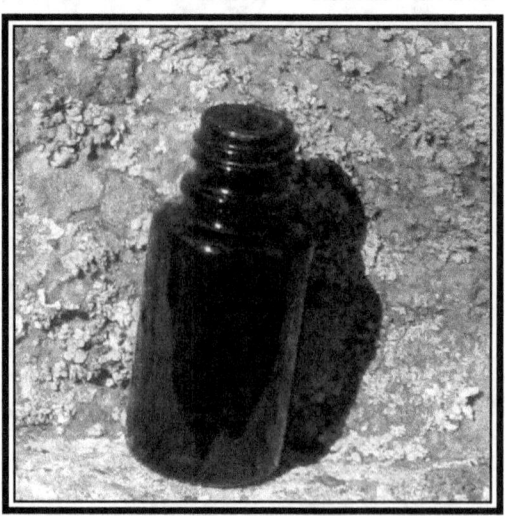

Myrtle Oil has a clear, herbaceous scent, which is very similar to eucalyptus essential oil.

It can be supportive of the respiratory system and encourages thyroid health.

Myrtle essential oil has soothing effects when inhaled, so it can be helpful for meditation and lifting the spirit.

Research has been done for its positive effects on glandular health challenges.

It is found in many skin and hair care products.

Nutmeg Oil has a spicy, warming aroma.

It has been used for culinary and medicinal purposes throughout history. As is true for many culinary oils, it can help with indigestion and support the digestive tract.

It can be supportive to the nervous and endocrine systems. Its revitalizing properties help to increase the body's energy.

Traditionally, it has been used to support normal circulation.

Tip: Use a drop of nutmeg essential oil when baking cookies to create a spicy, healthy treat.

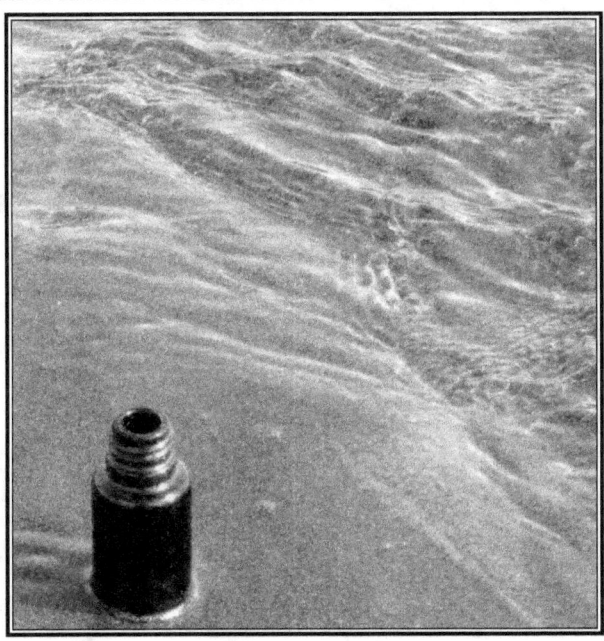

Orange Oil has a rich, citrus fruit scent that helps to lift up the spirit while providing a calming influence on the body. Orange essential oil is known to help bring peace and happiness to the mind.

It is rich in the powerful antioxidant d-limonene and can aid in maintaining normal cellular regeneration.

Pure, food grade orange essential oil may also be used when cooking to enhance the flavor of food.

Water or teas are more refreshing when a drop of orange essential oil is added.

Caution: As with after consuming most citrus fruits and oils, it is suggested you don't brush your teeth for at least 30 minutes after ingesting to protect tooth enamel.

Tip: Diffuse orange essential oil to lower anxiety, create a more positive mood and increase sleep time without fear of dampening general activity or motor coordination the next day.

Tip: To help with weight loss, add a few drops to a cold glass of plain or sparkling water to enjoy an energizing and refreshing drink and help relieve cravings for sugary or diet drinks.

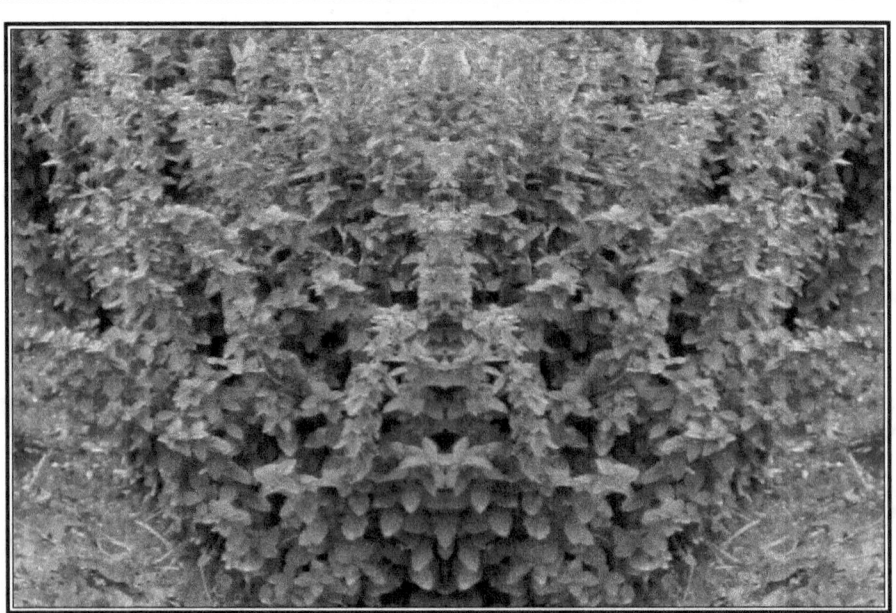

Oregano Oil has a pleasing scent that brings up memories of eating in an Italian restaurant.

Though most modern chefs think of its recipe potential, early uses were more medicinal than culinary.

Chinese doctors have used it to relieve fevers, vomiting, diarrhea, and itchy skin.

Europeans used it to sooth coughs and relieve indigestion.

Substitute oregano essential oil for various herbs when cooking and you and your family will benefit from its many therapeutic qualities.

It is a very powerful purifying and versatile essential oil.

Research reveals that it contains two essential components, thymol and carvacol, as does thyme. Thymol is beneficial for loosening phlegm in the lungs when one is very congested.

It can be used to enhance your immune system or support the respiratory system. It is touted for its antioxidant properties. Diffuse it during cold season to help reduce airborne bacteria in your home or office.

Massage it into tense muscles and joints to help them relax and release tension.

Tip: *When cooking an Italian meal, add some pure, food-grade oregano essential oil for healthy, authentic flavoring.*

Tip: *Used in tea, it can help relieve coughs or settle a queasy stomach.*

Tip: *Rub it on the bottom of your feet to relieve soreness and strengthen your immune system.*

Palo Santo Oil is one of Young Livings' exclusive essential oils that they have discovered and distill in Ecuador.

Traditionally, it has been used to ward off negative energies and protect one from negative spiritual influences.

Palo santo essential oil exhibits many properties similar to frankincense essential oil.

Patchouli Oil often brings back memories of "the sixties" with its musky, earthy, exotic aroma.

It is commonly used in Eastern cultures.

It can be used to provide general support for health and to help release negative emotions.

Patchouli essential oil can be used as a general tonic that supports the digestive system and soothes occasional queasiness.

When added to a carrier oil and applied topically, it can help smooth wrinkled skin or chapped appearance.

Tip: Diffuse it to relieve negative emotions and brighten your day.

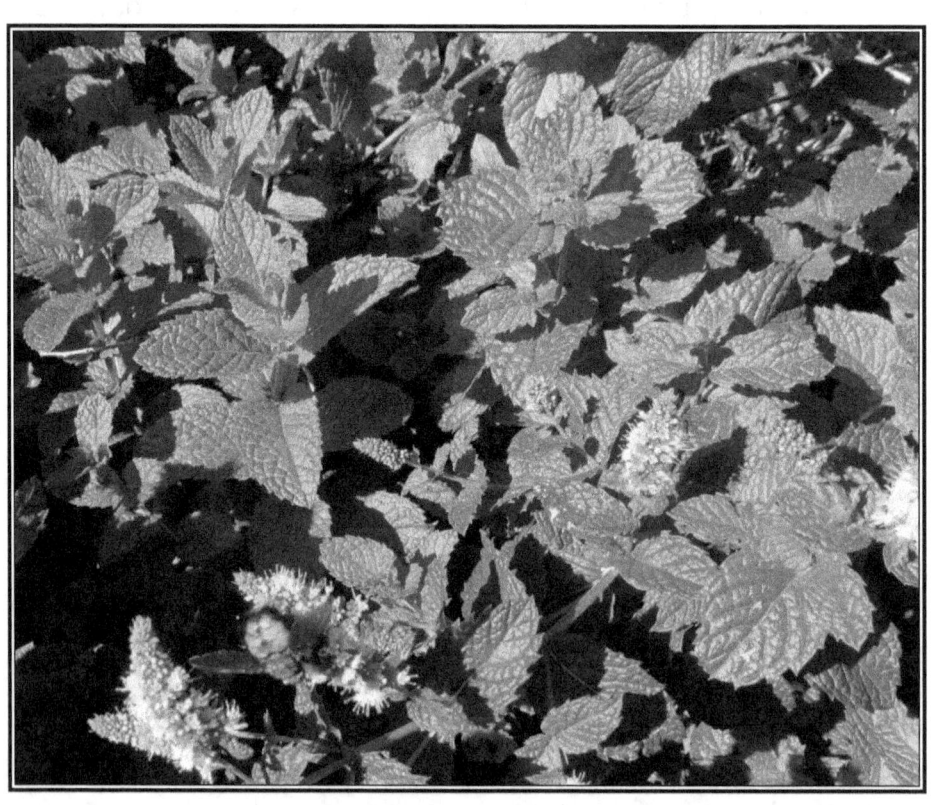

Peppermint Oil is another extremely versatile oil. It has a strong, clean, minty scent and can be used for many healthy purposes.

Every home should have a bottle of this wonderful essential oil.

Historically, it is one of the oldest herbs used for soothing digestion. Menthol is a potent aromatic chemical in the plants's volatile oil and is the active ingredient that gives peppermint essential oil its healing qualities.

It takes more to create therapeutic-grade peppermint essential oil than just finding the best plants.

When peppermint is harvested when the field's overall appearance goes from light to dark green; and the plant has just started to bloom before it is cut; and water is carefully measured prior to distillation, this will ensure that the most potent constituents are steam-extracted.

Peppermint essential oil stimulates the gallbladder and encourages bile secretion, as it helps the muscles of the stomach and intestines function more smoothly.

Scientists have researched peppermint's role in improving taste and smell when inhaled.

It can be used to enhance energy and fight off fatigue.

When inhaled, it helps improve concentration and increase mental sharpness.

Used in topical application for massage, you will experience the cooling sensation of menthol on overworked muscles or enjoy an invigorating foot scrub. Applied externally, it can relieve headaches and is good for rheumatism. It is a general stimulant to help bring the body back to its natural warmth in extreme cold.

Diffuse or directly breathe in its powerful aroma or make a tea to relieve congestion when suffering from a cold or the flu.

Peppermint essential oil tea is a wonderful soothing tea. It helps to cleanse and strengthen the entire body.

Put a drop in water instead of using a sugary after dinner mint. It will help freshen your breath and aid with digestion.

A cup of peppermint essential oil tea also offers headache relief. It helps strengthen the nerves instead of weakening them as aspirin and other drugs tend to do when used for pain or headaches.

It can be used when cooking or in baking to create healthy sweet treats.

Taken internally, it may help restore digestive efficiency or help curb appetites. Studies have shown it to directly affect the brain's satiety center, which triggers a sensation of fullness after meals. Any time of day, when added to your water it is very refreshing and helps curve cravings for sugary or diet drinks.

Or you can apply it topically to ease a queasy stomach.

Caution: Be careful to keep the oil away from your eyes.

Tip: Apply one or two drops (undiluted) just under your nose while driving in a car to keep your mind focused and help keep motion sickness symptoms under control.

Tip: To help relieve headaches, lie down and apply a drop on the temples or forehead, being careful to close your eyes, so there is no chance of it getting into your eyes.

Tip: To help aid in digestion, add a drop to herbal tea or massage several drops on the abdomen. You can place a drop on the tip of the tongue or wrists, or inhale to soothe minor stomach discomfort associated with travel.

Tip: Apply a drop or two to the back of your neck to help find relief from hot flashes.

Tip: Try spraying areas where ants or other insects enter your home with 15 drops of peppermint essential oil diluted in distilled water.

Tip: Place two drops on your tongue and rub another drop of oil under the nose to help improve concentration. Diffuse peppermint essential oil in areas when teaching to promote learning by your students.

Tip: To relieve a leg cramp, massage with peppermint essential oil.

Tip: Whenever you need to have an energy boost during the day, put a couple of drops of peppermint essential oil on the palms of your hand, rub them together, then hold them to your face and deeply breathe in the warm and invigorating scent. An added benefit, it has antibacterial properties, and if you are in a public setting it may aid in keeping any germs at bay.

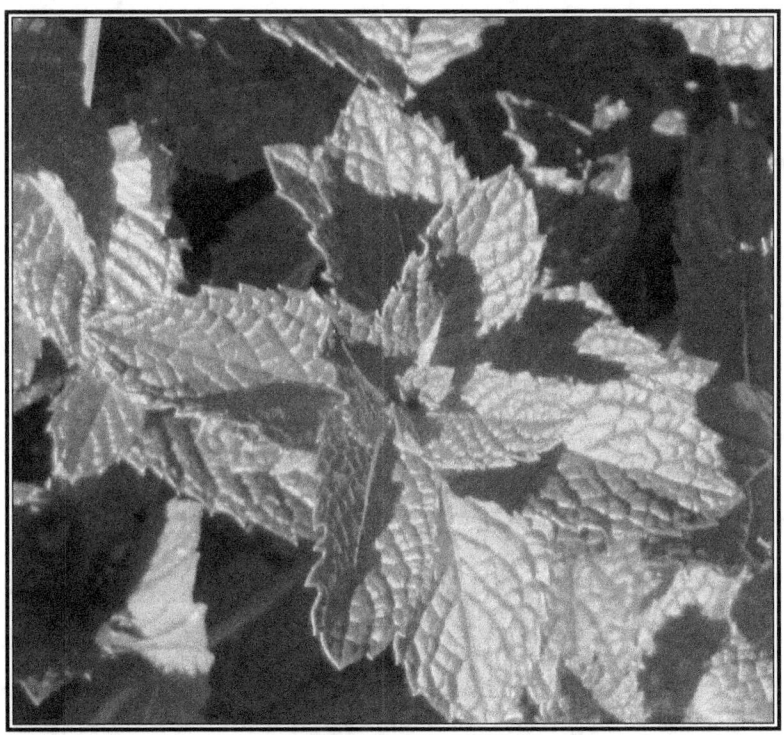

Fun Fact: The term "mint" is from the Greek name *Mintha*, a mythological nymph who was transformed into a plant by the goddess Persephone after she learned her husband Pluto was in love with her.

Pine Oil has an woodsy, refreshing, invigorating aroma and has an uplifting effect on the spirit and emotions. It has become one of my most favorite essential oils since originally writing this book.

It gives a home a fresh scent when used in cleaning or diffusing.

Pine essential oil will sooth stressed muscles and joints when used in massage.

Pine essential oil is a very powerful anti-inflammatory and very helpful to relieve the pain of arthritis.

It supports the respiratory system. It shares many of the same properties as eucalyptus globulus. The action of both essential oils is enhanced when they are blended.

Tip: Diffuse it to ward of negative emotions. Imagine taking a walk in a lovely pine forest and reset your attitude.

----------- ----------- ---------- ---------- ----------- ----------- ------------ ----------- ---------

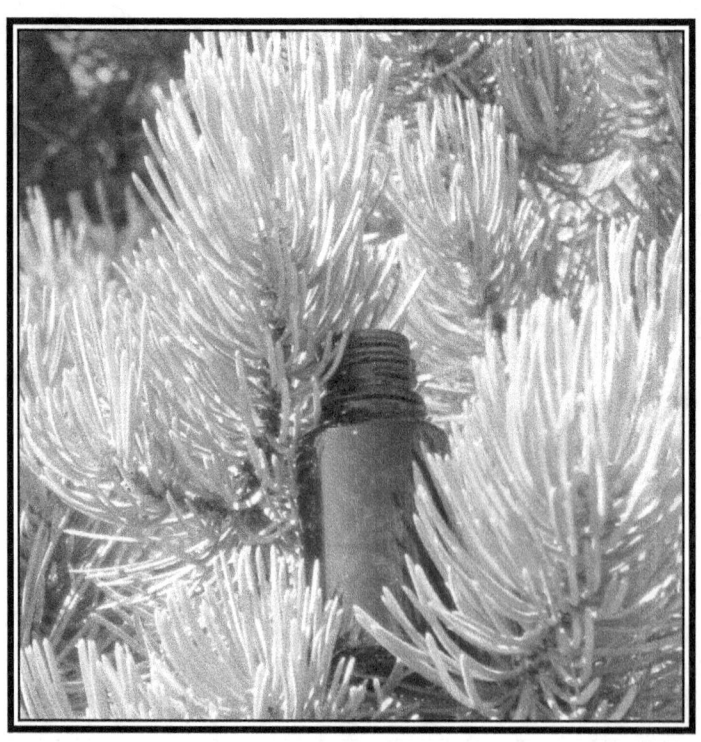

Rose Oil has a beautiful, strong floral fragrance that is very pleasant and is considered a highly romantic scent.

It can help bring balance and harmony to anyone's moods. Inhaling it helps reduce stress and nervousness.

Rose essential oil has been found to have a gentle balancing effect on hormone levels.

For thousands of years it has been used in skin care and it is very nourishing for dry or aging skin.

It is one of my, and many people's, most favorite aromas. When I walk in a room wearing it, often it seems to change the mood to a more happy place. Many people will comment upon how lovely the aroma is with a smile on their face.

Tip: *Rub rose essential oil over the heart area to lift a heavy mood and promote feelings of well-being and love.*

Tip: *Diffuse it before your special guest arrives in your home to create a romantic atmosphere.*

Tip: *Wearing rose essential oil everywhere you go evokes smiles and joy in other people.*

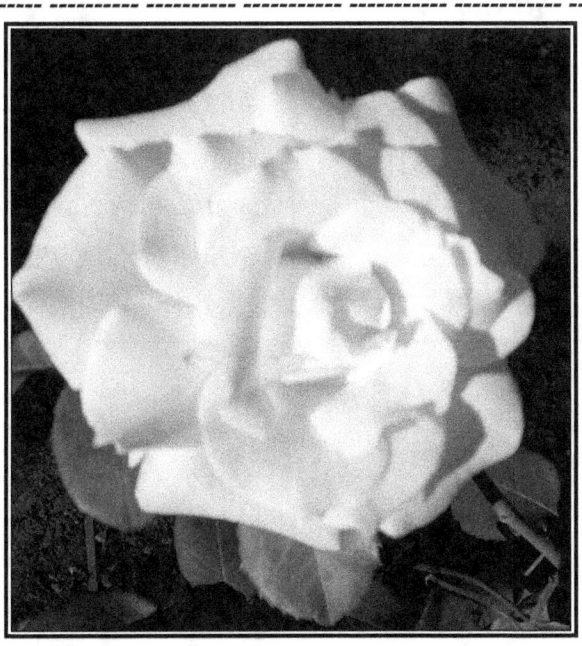

Rosemary Oil has a very strong, spicy, pine scent.

It is a strong antioxidant. It is considered a memory sharpener and can be inhaled directly or diffused to improve mental clarity and concentration.

Very good for headaches caused by nervousness. Inhale its aroma, or mix a bit in a carrier oil and rub it on the temples and the back of the neck for headache relief. *Caution: Keep it away from the eyes.*

As with many culinary herbs, rosemary essential oil has been used to soothe the digestive tract.

It aids in relaxing muscles and helps to relieve menstrual cramps.

Small amounts are as beneficial as larger doses, so use it sparingly when ingesting it. Always be sure you are using a 100% therapeutic-grade oil when consuming it.

Research is being done on how it may inhibit the growth and development of cancerous tumors in animals.

It is also found as an ingredient in hair care products.

Caution: **Large amounts of this oil may irritate the intestines.**

Caution: **Pregnant women should not use this oil medicinally.**

Tip: When cooking an Italian meal, add some pure, food-grade rosemary essential oil for healthy, authentic flavoring.

Tip: To add zest to the flavor of steamed vegetables. Put a drop or two of rosemary, basil, or thyme essential oils in the water.

Rosewood Oil has a lovely woody, lightly floral scent that is comforting and soothing.

It can have a steadying and balancing effect on emotions. It helps one to feel more grounded.

Inhaling rosewood essential oil can uplift feelings of deep sadness.

It is also used in skin care products and is very nourishing to the skin.

---------- ---------- ---------- ---------- ---------- ---------- ----------- ---------- ---------

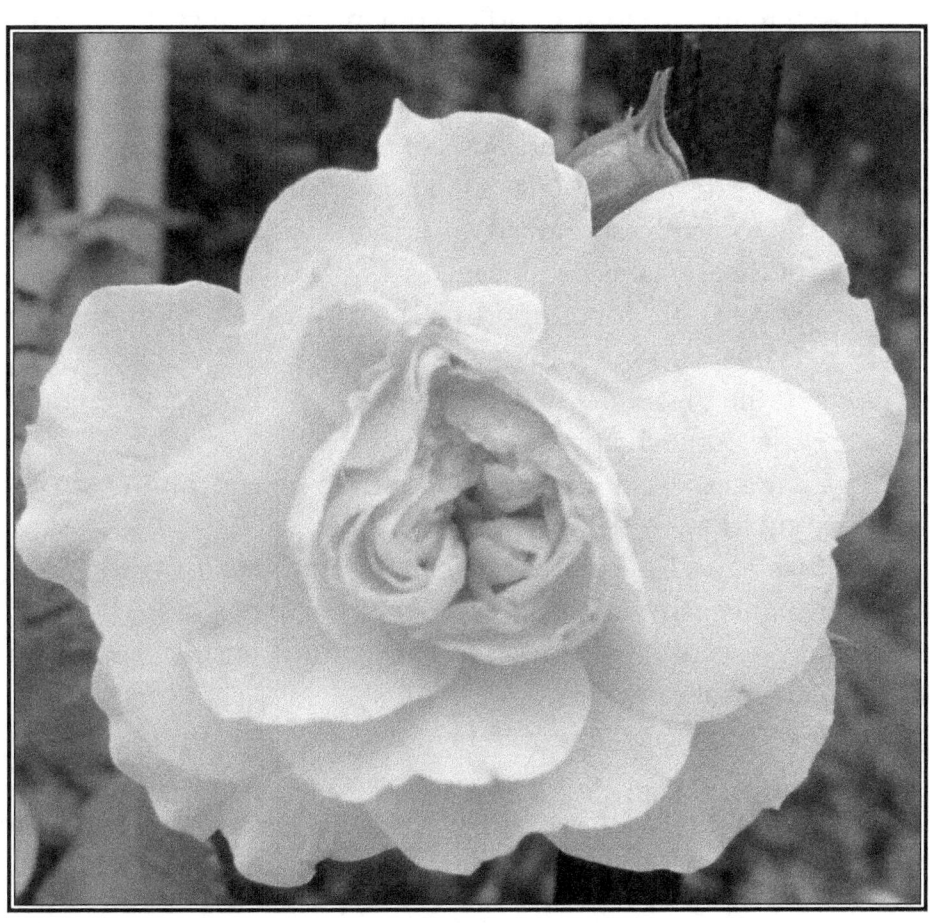

Sage Oil has a strong herbaceous aroma and is a very versatile oil.

It has been recognized for its ability to strengthen the senses and vital centers of the body. It can be used to support the body's metabolism.

Over the centuries, Greek's used sage essential oil for its varied medicinal properties. Historically, it has been used as a muscle relaxant, an antiperspirant and in skin care products.

Sage essential oil has been used for oral hygiene and as well as a treatment for sore throats.

It can also promote healing of wounds and insect bites.

In Europe it has been used traditionally for the skin.

It also may help to support a woman's natural cycles.

Sage tea is revered among the Chinese. They consider it as very soothing and quieting to the nerves, unlike black tea that can stress the nervous system.

Its antiseptic qualities make it a powerful healing agent when used topically or orally. Wounds of any kind will heal more rapidly if washed with sage essential oil tea.

It can be helpful for supporting the respiratory, reproductive, nervous, and other body systems.

One of the best remedies for stomach troubles, including gas in the stomach and bowels.

Use sage essential oil in a massage to help promote strong circulation.

Diffuse sage essential oil to cleanse and purify your home from negative influences. A deep breath of the aroma from sage essential oil may help in coping with despair and mental fatigue.

Hair care products use it to help alleviate dandruff.

Tip: For a sore throat, make a tea using a drop of pure sage essential oil. Let it cool. Gargle with it often.

Sandalwood Oil has a warm and woody aroma which is uplifting and relaxing. It is another "romantic" aroma and is considered to be very sensual.

Traditionally, throughout history, it is used as incense in religious ceremonies and to enhance the meditation experience by encouraging deeper concentration.

Similar to frankincense essential oil, it aids in supporting a healthy nervous and circulatory system. It is supportive of the body's natural defenses and helps support the body's immune system.

Sandalwood essential oil is highly valued in skin care products for its moisturizing and normalizing properties.

It is high in sesquiterpenes. It has been researched in Europe for its ability to oxygenate the part of the brain known as the pineal gland. This gland is responsible for releasing the hormone called melatonin, which enhances deep sleep.

Tip: Diffuse it before your special guest arrives in your home to create a romantic atmosphere.

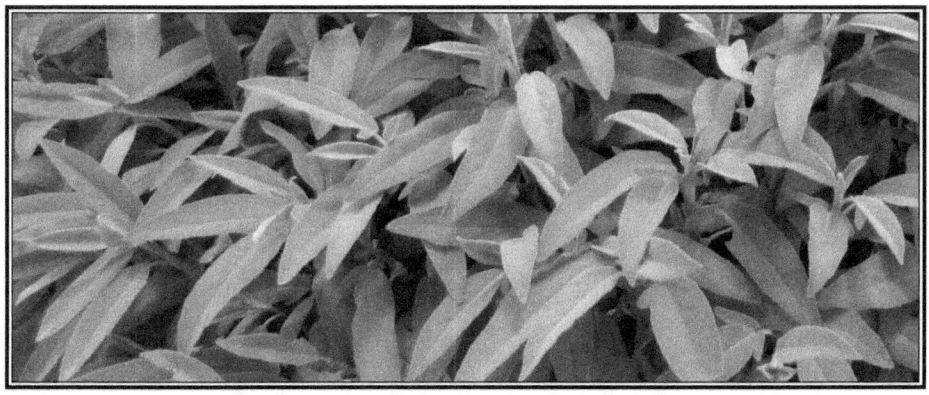

Spearmint Oil has a minty, slightly fruity scent, softer than peppermint essential oil.

Spearmint is rich in antioxidant menthol which makes it valuable in helping to support the respiratory and nervous systems.

Diffuse it or breathe it from the bottle to help open and release emotional blocks. This, in turn, will help a person gain a sense of emotional balance and well-being.

It is a highly regarded remedy for gas in the stomach and bowels and is useful when feeling nauseous and to stop vomiting. A cup of spearmint essential oil tea is a good way to quiet and soothe the stomach and jangled nerves.

Food-grade spearmint essential oil may also be used when cooking.

Or add a drop in hot tea or cold water for a refreshing beverage.

Tip: Add a few drops to a cold glass of water to deflect cravings for a sugary or diet drink.

Spruce Oil is similar to pine essential oil in scent and properties. It's aroma will make you think you are walking in a highly scented and peaceful forest.

It helps to support the respiratory system and can help relieve congested lungs.

Spruce essential oil will help to stimulate the immune system to ward off illnesses.

It is soothing to the nervous system and can be used in a massage to help relax tense muscles.

Its aromatic influences help to open and release emotional blocks to help bring about a feeling of balance and emotional well-being.

Native American Indians use it in ceremonies and regard it as a highly spiritual oil.

Tangerine Oil contains a powerful antioxidant, constituent d-limonene.

Use tangerine essential oil to support the bodys' natural defenses and encourage healthy digestion.

Diffuse its sweet citrus fragrance to elicit feelings of happiness and wellness.

Tip: Try adding a couple of drops to a cup of tea to sooth a troubled stomach.

Tip: Add a few drops to a cold glass of water to deflect cravings for a sugary or diet drink.

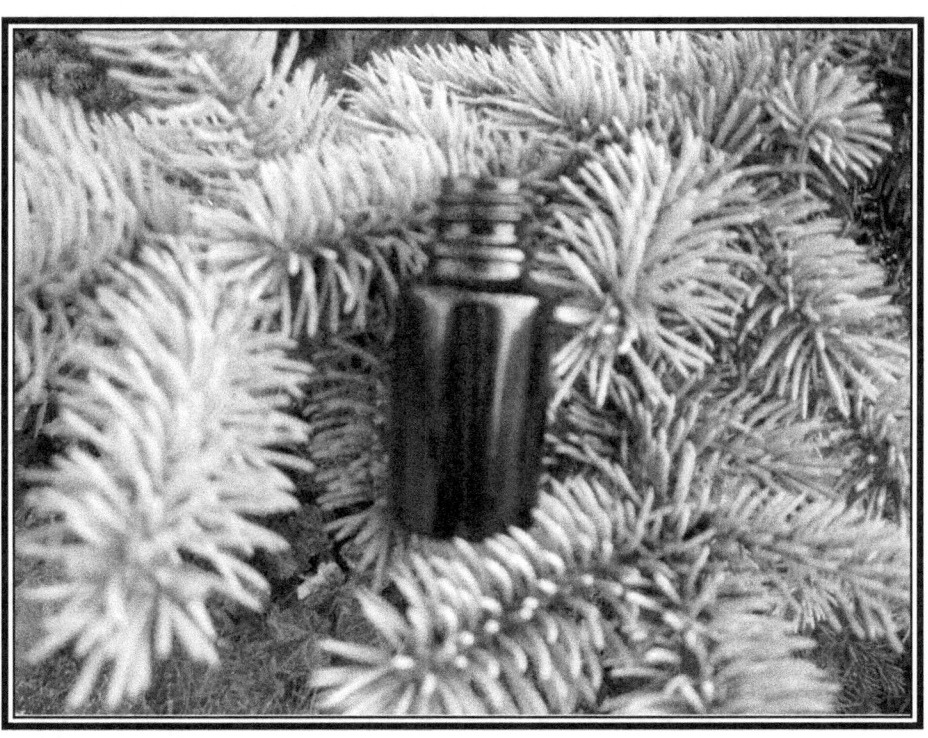

Tarragon Oil is another essential oil that has been revered for its culinary and medicinal qualities for centuries in many cultures.

Use it to soothe and support the digestive system.

It can be helpful in overcoming the flu.

It may have the ability to cleanse the body of free radicals. Research is being done on its potential for blocking cancer.

Tip: When cooking an Italian meal, add pure, food-grade tarragon essential oil for healthy, authentic flavoring.

----------- ----------- ---------- ---------- ----------- ----------- ------------ ----------- ---------

Thyme Oil has a warm, spicy, herbaceous aroma that is both powerful and penetrating.

Since ancient times, thyme essential oil has been used as both a culinary and a medicinal herb.

As a dietary supplement, it is one of the strongest antioxidants.

Thyme essential oil can be used to support the immune, respiratory, digestive, nervous, and other body systems.

It can also relieve headache pain.

Thyme essential oil has antibacterial and antifungal properties.

When ingested or inhaled, it helps loosen phlegm and relax the muscles of the respiratory system. It helps to relieve coughs resulting from colds, bronchitis and emphysema. Put a drop or two in steaming water and deeply breathe in to relieve congested nose and lungs.

Food-grade thyme essential oil may also be used when cooking to create healthy and flavorful dishes.

Caution: Too large a dose of thyme essential oil can cause intestinal problems. As this is a very strong oil, always dilute thyme when ingesting or massaging it into your body.

Tip: Add zest to the flavor of steamed vegetables. Put a drop or two of rosemary, basil, or thyme essential oil in the water you are using to steam the vegetables.

Tip: When cooking an Italian meal, add thyme essential oil for healthy, authentic flavoring.

----------- ----------- ---------- ---------- ----------- ----------- ------------ ----------- ---------

Valerian Oil is distilled from valerian root.

Valerian has been used for thousands of years for its calming, grounding, and emotionally balancing influences.

Valerian essential oil is considered a safe aid to sleep. It helps calm anxiety and has sedative, sleep-enhancing properties when inhaled.

During the last three decades, it has been clinically investigated for its relaxing properties.

Researchers have pinpointed the sesquiterpenes, valerenic acid, and valerone as the active constituents that exert a calming and restorative effect on the central nervous system.

Studies show it helps people with insomnia fall asleep faster; sleep better and longer; and awake feeling refreshed; a powerful antioxidant not groggy in the morning.

Interesting Fact: Valium is a prescription drug sedative and has no relationship to valerian.

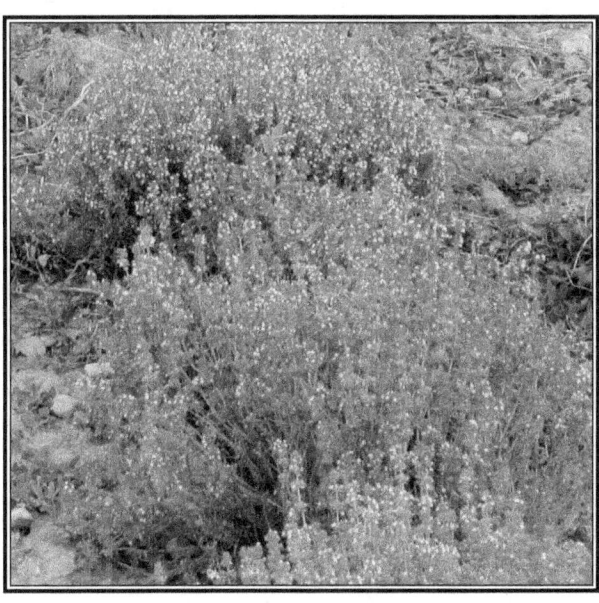

Vetiver Oil has a similar aroma to patchouli essential oil.

It is one of the essential oils that is very high in sesquiterpenes.

Traditionally, it is used for relaxation and easing anxiety. It helps psychologically ground and calm you and aid in regaining a sense of emotional well-being.

Diffuse vetiver essential oil to help cope with stress or recover from an emotional shock or trauma.

Research has shown it to improve children's behavior.

Topically it can be beneficial in cleansing a wound and promote healing.

---------- ----------- --------- ---------- ----------- ---------- ------------ ---------- ---------

Wintergreen Oil has a minty scent that reminds one of the winter holidays.

This oil is distilled from the small evergreen herb's leaves. It contains natural methyl salicylae, which is highly regarded for its soothing properties for stressed muscles and head tension.

The refreshing, clean taste of wintergreen has made it a favorite in flavoring numerous products.

Wintergreen essential oil is beneficial in massage for soothing head tension and muscles after exercising.

Wintergreen essential oil tea is beneficial as a gargle for a sore throat and mouth and leaves your breath feeling fresh.

It may help relieve chronic inflammatory rheumatism.

Tip: Massage wintergreen essential oil into the feet at night to relieve foot pain after a long exercise session or hike.

---------- ----------- --------- ---------- ----------- ---------- ------------ ---------- ---------

Ylang Ylang Oil has a soft, flowery fragrance that for centuries has made it a romantic favorite.

Ylang Ylang essential oil can be extremely effective in calming and bringing about a sense of relaxation.

Diffuse it to help with releasing nervous tension or relieve irritability.

Inhale it using deep, slow breaths when feeling anger or frustration to help release and redirect these emotions.

Ylang Ylang essential oil has a long history of use in skin care and hair products that promote luxuriant, healthy hair.

Tip: Diffuse it to create a more romantic atmosphere in the bedroom for a night of romance.

Tip: Add to food or rice milk as a dietary supplement or for flavoring.

---------- ---------- ---------- ---------- ---------- ---------- ----------- ---------- ---------
---------- ---------- ---------- ---------- ---------- ---------- ----------- ---------- ---------
---------- ---------- ---------- ---------- ---------- ---------- ----------- ---------- ---------

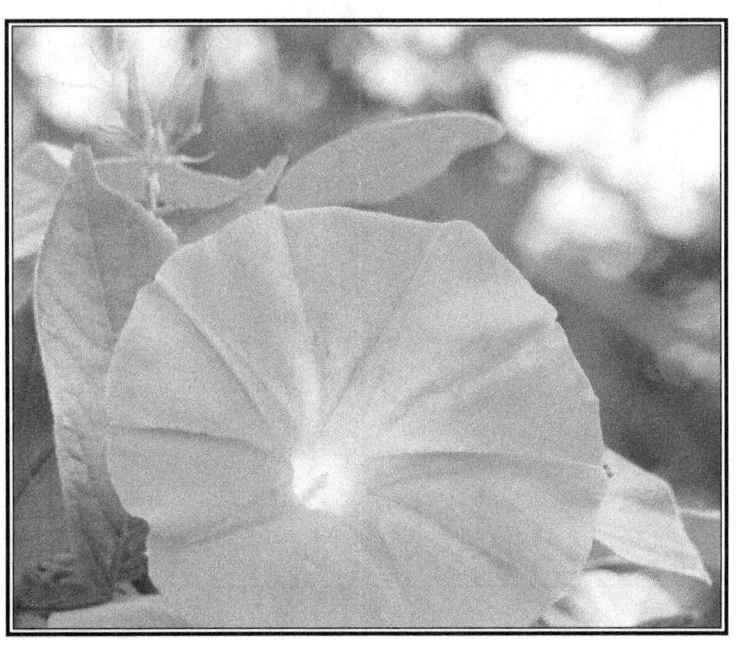

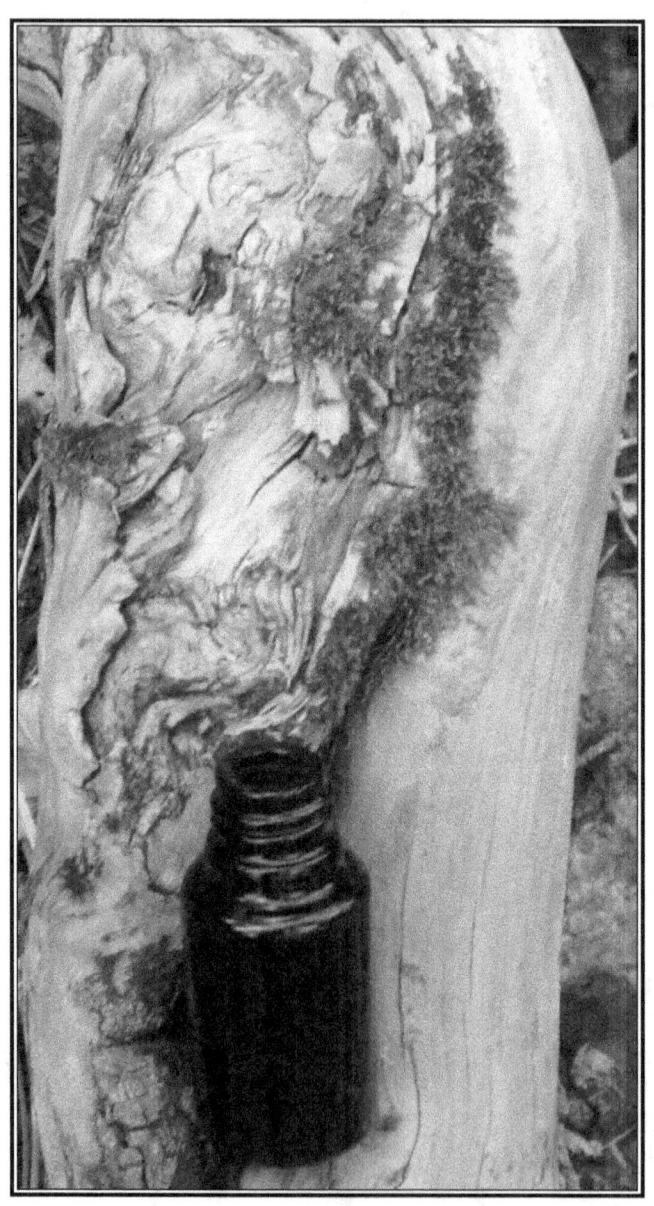

AFTERWORDS

These tips and informative descriptions found in this book come directly from a Young Living Essential Oils distributor and are passed on to you using her knowledge base. The company and author assumes no liability for any damage caused by use of these Tips.

---------- --------- --------- ---------- ----------- ------------ ----------

Using Essential Oils has Helped many People Step on the (W)right Path to Optimum Health and Invite Abundance into their Lives.

Take Your First Step to Experiencing Natural Optimum Health TODAY!

---------- --------- --------- ---------- ----------- ------------ ----------

By searching the web, you can learn many more ways to create natural, positive healing conditions and optimum health for you and your family when using essential oils.

Try searching the internet using the name of an essential oil that interests you to discover other helpful tips and historical pieces of information about specific (aromatic) essential oils you think you might enjoy using or learning more about.

Or visit my blog at:
www.usingessentialoils.com.

Essential Oil Name	Calming / Relaxing	Uplift Spirits / Balance	Energizing	Circulation / Heart	Mental Alertness	Digestive / Elimination	Respiratory / Decongesting	Immune System	Anti-infections	Relax Muscles	Pain / Headache Relief	Anti-Aging	Hormonal Balance	Supports Nervous System
Balsam Fir	X	X		X		X				X	X			
Basil			X	X	X					X				
Bergamot	X	X			X	X				X				
Cedarwood	X	X			X		X			X	X			
Chamomile (Ger)	X	X				X			X	X	X			
Cinnamon Bark		X	X			X	X	X	X					
Citronella			X						X	X	X		X	
Clary Sage	X	X								X	X	X	X	
Clove			X			X	X	X	X		X	X		
Coriander		X		X	X	X				X	X		X	
Cypress	X	X		X	X					X	X			
Dill	X					X		X	X					
Elemi								X	X		X	X		
Eucalyptus		X	X	X			X		X	X	X			
Eucalyptus Blue							X							
Frankincense	X	X					X			X	X	X		X
Geranium	X	X		X		X				X			X	
Ginger		X	X			X			X	X	X			
Grapefruit		X	X					X	X					
Helichrysum	X	X		X						X				
Hyssop	X			X			X	X	X					X
Jasmine	X	X											X	
Juniper		X	X			X	X							X
Lavender	X	X	X	X	X	X			X	X	X			X
Lemon			X	X		X	X	X	X	X		X		
Lemongrass	X	X		X	X	X		X	X		X	X		X

Essential Oil Name	Calming/Relaxing	Uplift Spirits/Balance	Energizing	Circulation/Heart	Mental Alertness	Digestive/Elimination	Respiratory/Decongesting	Immune System	Anti-infections	Relax Muscles	Pain/Headache Relief	Anti-Aging	Hormonal Balance	Supports Nervous System
Marjoram	X			X		X			X	X	X			
Melaleuca							X	X	X	X				
Melissa	X	X						X	X			X		
Mountain Savory		X	X		X			X	X	X				
Myrrh	X	X						X	X				X	X
Myrtle	X	X					X	X		X				
Nutmeg		X	X	X		X		X					X	X
Orange & Tangerine	X	X				X			X	X		X		
Oregano		X		X		X	X	X	X	X	X			X
Palo Santo	X	X						X		X	X	X		
Patchouli	X	X				X		X						
Peppermint		X	X	X	X	X	X	X	X	X	X			X
Pine		X	X					X		X	X			
Rose	X	X												X
Rosemary	X	X												
Rosewood					X			X			X			
Sage	X	X	X		X	X	X	X	X	X	X	X	X	
Sandalwood	X	X		X					X	X	X			X
Spearmint		X				X	X							
Spruce		X	X					X	X		X			X
Tarragon	X					X		X						X
Thyme							X	X	X	X	X	X		
Valerian	X	X												X
Vetiver	X	X							X	X			X	X
Wintergreen		X	X							X	X			
Ylang Ylang	X	X		X						X			X	

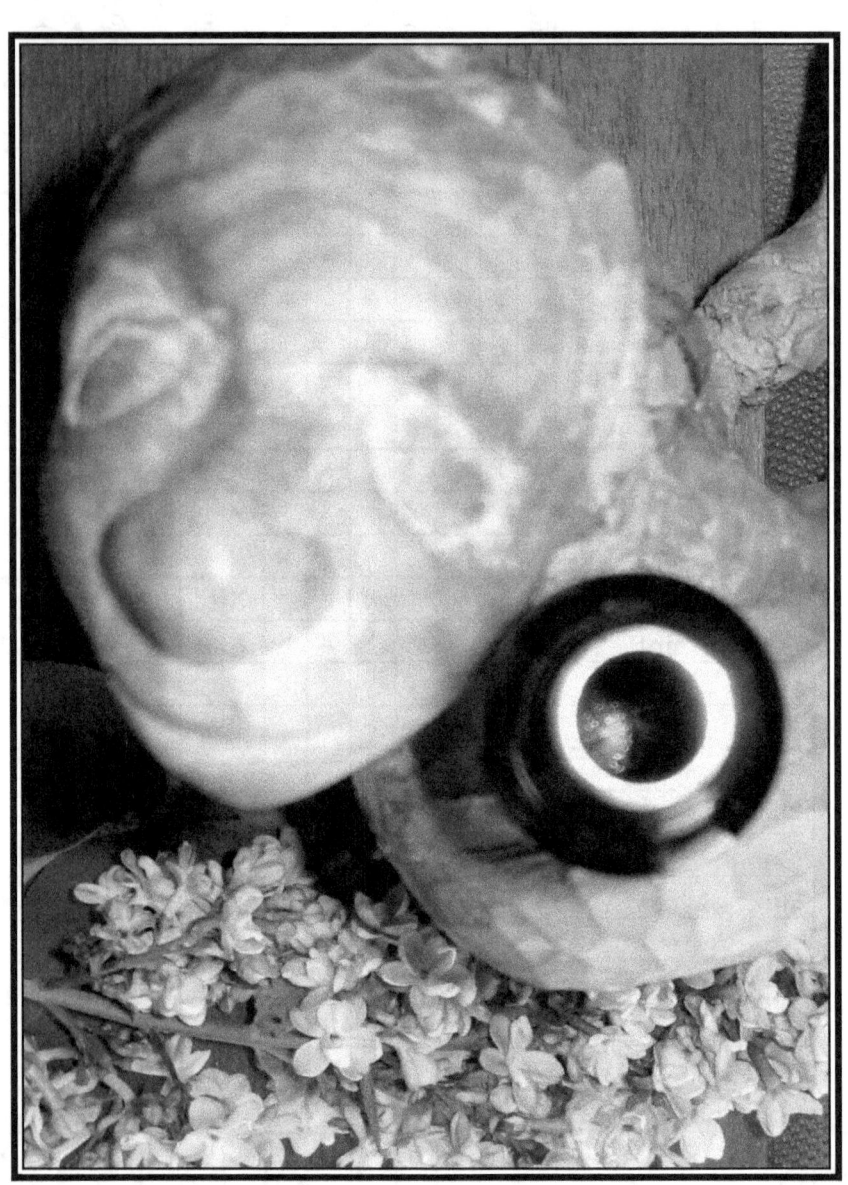

Epilogue

An Invitation to Share

Please take a moment to share any great results you have achieved in using essential oils, so others might gain some insights for dealing with health challenges or how to start living in a more natural and healthy environment.

Please email and let me know which of the essential oils *"Tips"* in this book you found most useful.

I would invite you to email your essential oils usage tips and healing stories, along with your name and city to:

info@usingessentialoilsforhealth.com.

Please be aware that by sending us your tips, you are granting us permission to publish them and post them on the internet in our blog, as well as to edit them for length, mechanics and content.

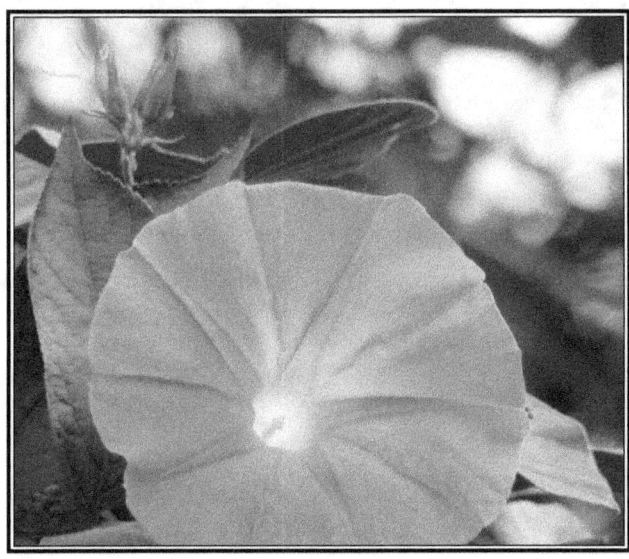

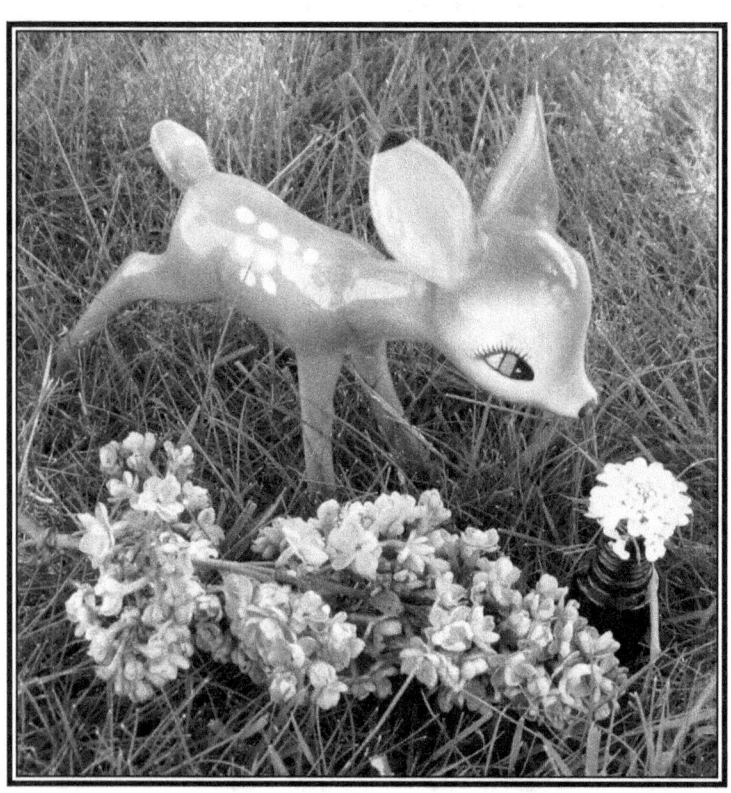

About the Author

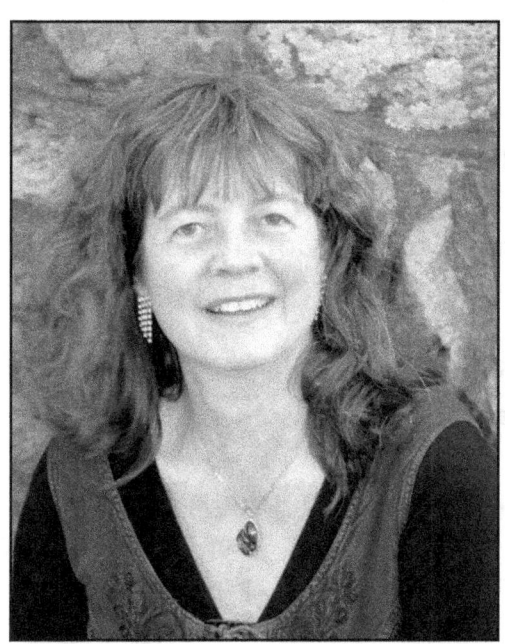

Julia L. Wright has been using essential oils for over 19 years and has many success stories to share about how they work to help regain or maintain optimum health.

Julia is an author and artist who lives in a small Colorado mountain town at the foot of Pikes Peak. Here artists, environmentalists, and holistic healers abound.

Many years ago she discovered there are many different ways to integrate essential oils into a person's healing path.

Recently she began sharing ways to live a more holistic life, including using essential oils, at www.HolisticSteps.com. Visit here to read more true life stories about how she has integrated essential oils into her daily life.

Over the past 19 years, she has used many different essential oils to help overcome various health challenges she has experienced.

Kathleen Morrow, Julia's good friend, an aromatherapist and a Craniosacral Therapist, has taught her many ways to use essential oils beginning when Julia was recovering from a car accident. The accident left Julia with many physical pains and a "slight" concussion, causing a mental and emotional shift. Julia used various essential oils to stimulate her brain in positive ways and help relieve painful muscles.

About 13 years ago, Julia had a minor surgery that gave her a major complication. She developed a blood clot that almost filled her left venous vein.

She spent 10 days in the hospital and was sent home with a leg that was hugely swollen and many "lovely" shades of purple.

A nurse described the problem as having a *"killer "* in her leg.

She could barely walk and had to use a cane and lift her leg up when climbing stairs. She spent most of her days with it elevated.

Three different doctors told her she would have to live with this health challenge and they couldn't help her in any way. These doctors also wanted her to remain on Coumadin (a blood thinner) for the rest of her life! *Who would want to be using "rat poison" for "healing" for the rest of their life?*

Julia wanted to stabilize this huge blood clot, but her body did not like Coumadin at all. Her body would flush it out or not use it in a way that would show up with the proper number in the blood samples. The technician was unable to stabilize the dosage. The technician would order her to take a higher and higher dose each week, until it reached a level that even had him nervous. She quickly fired all those doctors. After just six months, when she felt comfortable that the clot was stabilized, she began using only totally natural approaches to dissolve the clot. The hospital nurse had given her the best information about what was going on in her leg and what she needed to be aware of before letting go of that dangerous drug in order to avoid causing a worse health challenge.

Julia worked with her long-time General Practitioner (GP) and a renowned holistic healer (Vivian Rice) during those first six months. They helped her to find the way to step on a path to a totally natural approach to resolving this health challenge and begin her journey back to optimum health.

Part of the journey included taking short walks every day, that would lengthen as her leg improved. Now she takes longer hikes, sometimes for miles on weekends, or walks somewhere in town every day. Four years after that dire diagnosis, she hiked 13 mountainous miles in five hours.

Over the years, Julia has reduced this major complication to a slight inconvenience. She continues to use many essential oils to keep herself as healthy as possible naturally.

Even her GP was amazed at the progress she made in the first year and as long as she worked with her. She encouraged Julia every step of the way back to a gaining a healthier leg and body.

Julia has used many natural supplements, essential oils, craniosacral therapy, massage, acupuncture and exercises to get her life back to a semblance of normality after every health challenge that has come her way. Essential oils have been integrated into every part of her life to create her optimum health.

Every night and morning, she massages her legs, feet and neck with a variety of Young Living essential oils and oil blends. This massage time may include lavender, geranium, peppermint, pine, cypress, cedarwood, helichrysum and AromaLife™. These various essential oils help to keep the circulation in her leg healthy, rebuild tissue and keep the bruised areas and swelling to a minimum.

She also uses Young Living essential oil blends called Valor™ and Harmony™ help to keep her mood uplifted.

Julia continues to use a combination of single essential oils and oil blends to help relieve pain caused by the car accident when she experiences them in various parts of her body.

In this book, Julia invites you to take the first step on your path to safely regaining and maintaining your optimum health by integrating essential oils into your daily health regime.

More Resources:

Learn how to purchase Young Living Essential Oils or become a distributor by going to www.youngliving.org/juliaw.

Kathleen Morrow, RCST®, RPP, LMT, teaches classes to relating to using essential oils and the Raindrop Therapy at the School of Inner Health in Colorado Springs, Colorado. Check it out if you are looking to learn a new healing technique at:
www.sharinginnerhealth.com.

Vivian Rice is a renowned Nutritionalist in Colorado Springs, CO. Simple dietary changes to help you and your family find a way to Optimum health can be found at:
www.HandbooktoHealth.com.

Notes

Notes

Notes

Notes

Notes